MARKETING Secrets

I would like to dedicate this book to my Inspired members, who have been apart of the inspired online program. They have actually been my true inspiration and I have so much love for each of them. I am delighted to watch as they realise their own potential. It's like being a very proud mother to over six hundred children, and I hope to continue to grow my family and be wowed at the things these fantastic techs do for the industry.

A heart felt thank you.

I would also like to dedicate this book to my mentors, I have invested in my own education and without their guidance and support, I am not sure I would have had the confidence to write this book. You know who you are, thankyou.

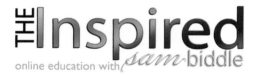 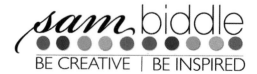

www.sambiddle.online : beinspired@sambiddle.co.uk
Cover Design by #MOMBOSS Digital Marketing Jenny Allen

Table of Contents

You did a good thing!

Congratulations for buying this book.

Firstly I want to say thank you for buying this book, so you're either a nail technician, beauty therapist or hairdresser, it literally doesn't matter what you do, I am going to assume it's your business to make your clients look and feel good every day.

Right, so now we have established that you have picked up the right book Let me ask you, how is your turnover?

Do you understand your cash flow and what your profit margins are with each treatment you offer? No? Then you and I need to talk.

Because it's not ok to be just a nail tech, beauty therapist or hair stylist, you're a businessperson and running a business is no joke, if you haven't already realised it. In business you need to wear many different hats.

Now don't panic, this is not a book on profit and losses and has zero accountancy speak, but I want to talk to you about the second most important thing when it comes to being in business and that is marketing.

Having been marketing myself and my business for the nearly "cough" 30 years. Way before Facebook and the phenomenon which is social media. I had to meet people face to face to get new customers. But you're lucky, we now live in a social media society and it is a fabulous way to get your business in front of your new clients.

In this book and the course that supports it, I will teach you how to target your customers, find out who they are, what they want from you and develop a message they understand and get excited by. I will also show you how to build your own profile and a voice your clients will listen to. The difference between Instagram and Facebook and where to find those elusive clients.

This book is about marketing for nail professionals, beauty therapists and hair stylists who run their own business's or are starting out. But if I am honest, the message is the same regardless of what type of creative or artistic business your in. Just swap out the words clients for customer and salon for studio.

You see marketing is a form of storytelling, and a creative process in its self, but too many times I see my fellow business persons (alittle PC goes a long way!) shy away from it. I hope I can show you it is a fun thing to do and not something to procrastinate over.

Regardless of how creative we are, we need to remember that we are in business, and if we want to continue to enjoy our creative employment we have to learn the subtle art of marketing. So how is it that I can talk to you about this expansive topic?

Having manipulated words to create stories about the things I sell, so people want to buy them, from the time before social media, I started refining my marketing nohow by selling pottery! Yes you heard me, Pottery! Then it was electricity to tattoo's, tanning and nail art. But in truth, I have learned to adapt my skills and using it to sell my passions. Yes it is that simple and I will show you how in this book.

Very aware of the need for speed, the chapters in this book are short and concise, giving you the information you need today without the fluff.

This book is designed to deliver all the marketing no how you can refer back to. I hope you can take away some useful hints, tips and nuggets of pure gold which you can cash in at the bank and make all your hard work worthwhile.

Even though we've made it our vocation to enhance peoples lives with beauty, colour and touch, we are, after all in business and need to pay our own rent.

I would like to say thank you and well done for picking up this book, and taking ownership of the magnificent world of marketing, it's one of the best parts of my job and I hope you fall in love ith it as well.

This book is just the starting point, and the tip of a rather larger marketing iceberg. If you want to know more after reading this, get intouch with me, I have a wealth of great people I can recommend to follow on social.

One last thing, I want to leave you with, marketing should be considered an art form, it is only through being creative that you can enjoy the full benefits of this beautiful craft.

Who is Sam Biddle.

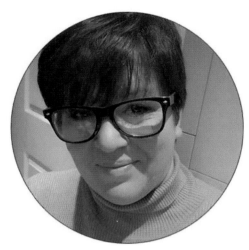

This is where I need to write the 'How did you get to where you are?' blurb. Those who know me and have attended any of my classes, will know my 'about me' speech is always something I struggle with, but this is a book on marketing and the first rule I will teach you is that people buy from people. So I suppose you should know who I am.

At 47 I find myself in a rather idyllic situation, working from home, in a small office with a fabulous assistant and being able to run two international companies.

Be Inspired is my baby and is all about education and self-development. Be Creative is Co-owned with my business partner Rebecca Orme and a product-led company which offers unique and innovative nail art solutions. Call me a rule breaker, many do, and I don't care, because for the past 18 years bending and challenging the industries norms has been rather fun. Playing with additives was once a rarity for a tech and raised a few eyebrows in the past, but 5 years ago I introduced my pigments. My philosophy is that no matter how mad you think an idea is, try it, experiment and see what magic you can make. There is always a way!

I started in the nail industry by accident; I used to buy little kits from QVC. Obsessed with nail art, little did I know then, in October 1999 that I would do what I do now.

A nail technician and salon owner, I was probabaly just like you, working 7 days a week with two children, it very nearly killed me. No joke…I diced with the Big C!

I realised I needed to find a secret superpower to leverage my time and still earn money.

This was all before social media and the wonders of facebook.

Moving into education and developing my online courses, I found the something even sexier than a superpower.

I made marketing my Bitch!

Yep, I defiantly made mistakes and lost a ton of money, wasted time on things that just didn't work and missed out on opportunities. But as soon as I learned the art of marketing, everything changed.

But let us go back in time, so you can get the low down on who wrote this book.

In July 2007 after a few bumps on my nail journey, I started Be Inspired. I wanted to provide learning and education for designs that were unique and different but could be incorporated into the brand that each individual nail technician knows and loves. I was an educator for EzFlow Nail Systems and I wanted to concentrate on my passion for teaching, not having the salon to divide my time I attended college to undertake my teaching certificate.

Be Inspired was growing into an international success story, I developed four classes which would help technicians to find inspiration and express their creativity. I was the first Independent Educator in the UK and although we see a fair few around now; I feel I still offer the industry something different through my education activities.

If I am honest applying nails is a by-product, being a nail tech allows me to develop structure and control the creative flow, it provides mini canvases with which to paint on and gives me the revenue to enjoy my job but it is the art which keeps me going, this is a tough industry.

But what turns me on, is business, yes you guessed it, marketing!

Writing and releasing my first book "The secret to great nail art" in 2017, sparked a desire for writing. It is a workbook for nail artists to support my signature course Be Inspired online for life.

I have been fortunate to have worked with some amazing titles, from Cosmopolitan magazine and Woman to attending photo shoots and working with supermodels. Having a 4 page spread in the Independent and a centre spread in the Daily Mail featuring my extreme nail art designs, plus filming for Sky Living. There have been some interesting experiences throughout my career and I am trying to remember them all, the highlights have to be my fantasy images being used for the 2012 Nailympia advertising campaign, My Nail Talk Radio interview in the USA, Being an international judge for NailPro (2010-2014) And being invited as an international judge for Nailympia 2013, 2015, 2017,2018. Achieving front covers in many trade magazines and being a columnist for Scratch magazine and Professional nails, I look back on my career and think, wow, never in a million years, when I bought that little nail art kit from QVC did I imagine all this.

Phew, now that the name dropping is out of the way, let me explain why I wrote this little book.

This is a sexy subject, trust me. But really I wrote this book to answer the many questions I get asked about marketing, social media and business. Regardless of how creative we are, we need to remember that we are in business and if we want to continue to enjoy this creative employment; we have to learn the subtle art of marketing. So how is it I can mark these pages with words on this expansive topic?

Having been in business for myself since I was 19 years old (basically, I have never had a "real job" as my father-in-law likes to call it.) I have manipulated words to sell, creating a story people listen to, enjoy and then buy. Basically, that is all marketing is. From the time before social media, I refined my marketing no-how by selling everything from pottery, electricity to tattoos, tanning, and nail art. Now "they" call it internet entrepreneurism but in fact, I have learned to adapt my skills and use them to sell my passions, moving through the years to refine my skills I have learned.

Very aware of the need for speed, the chapters in this book are short and concise, giving you the information you need today without the fluff.

This book is your introduction into Marketing, the first step you need to get started.

Enjoy, and let me know what you think.
Sam

People buy from people.

Marketing is not everyone's cup of tea but it is an important part of being in business.

It doesn't matter if you are the hottest nail artist, the best therapist or whackiest hair stylist in town if you don't have enough clients to keep you in business!

If you understand marketing then you will outgrow those that don't master the basics and understand this beautiful creative craft.

What is Marketing?

Marketing is the process of teaching clients why they should choose you over your competitors. The key is finding the right message which will influence the decision to choose you and comes back for repeat business.

The mistake is thinking marketing is just "one" thing, but marketing is everything that the client encounters when they come to your salon, from advertising, to what they hear, to the customer service they receive, to the follow-up care you provide.

Imagine your reading a beautiful romance. A young girl is being courted by the handsome boy, wooed and wowed, she eventually agrees to go on a date. He takes her to a beautiful restaurant, and she is all dressed up and expecting wonderful things. He ends up kissing her on the doorstep, after a few months of dating, he bends down on one knee and proposes. Riding off into the sunset they live happily ever after.

Come on now, don't deny it, you have all read at least one trashy chick lit romance, I will be honest with you, I much prefer my books to be a tad more steamy with shades of grey, but for now this is a great example.

Imagine you're the writer of this book. You're weaving a story between a couple falling in love. You can decide where the story goes, you're developing the characters and getting to know who they are and what they like.

Marketing is exactly like that. You have a business and you need to find a client- you need to court them until they want to marry you and live happily ever after.

Too many times my students will say;
        "well I posted a photo of my nails, and got no likes, so marketing doesn't work for me."
I ask them how often they posted and what did they say to attract the customer, more often than not there is a blank stare. "My work should speak for its self." They say.

If a guy came up to you and said: "I look good so you should marry me." How would you react?

Marketing is a dance, a courtship between you and someone you have not met yet. Your job is to provide them with the information they need to find you attractive enough to pay attention.

Selling to your peers and not your customers.

Social media is a fantastic place to build communities of technicians, therapists and stylists. Coming from the nail industry I know there are many groups to support professionals and encourage their ideas and growth when it comes to application.

But what I also see, is a lot of those technicians forget who their real customers are. They spend a lot of their time showing off their work to their peers and not selling them to their customers. Your peers might give you compliments which boosts your self-esteem, but does not boost your bank account. Don't worry about what your peers are doing or saying, market to your clients, think about what they want!

Customers are not sitting in these professional groups and it is important to target your ideal customer. Just like any courtship you have a type, and that type likes to hang out in his or her favourite place.

Figuring out who your new clients are, where they hang out and what they like, is the first step towards building your marketing plan.

Who is your audience?

I will call it an audience because you're now performing in front of these potential clients and delivering a message.
But you don't want a crowd of die-hard, heavy metal fans coming to an opera. They won't enjoy the show. So making sure you invite the right people to hear the things they can relate to or enjoy is key to making your marketing work.

Start by asking yourself some simple questions.

What problems do you solve? You should have some understanding of why your product or service exists. If you're a hair stylist, then you know the main issue people have is their hair gets long. Nail technicians can help clients with their short, untidy nails and so forth.
Who are our current clients? How far do they travel to get to you, how much do they spend, what is the most popular service you provide?
Who is your competition? It's likely you know who your obvious competitors are. However, some quick searches on Google and social media can often reveal competition you may not have known of. Try searching for a keyword or two that relates to your industry. See which businesses come up. Browse their "About Us" pages and feature descriptions. This is an easy way to develop an idea of who your competition is.
What do customers stand to gain from choosing you? What features do you offer that no one else does? Is there something you can do better than anyone else? This is called your unique selling point (USP)

I will be going deeper into this subject later on in the book, where we work out who your ideal client is and more importantly how to speak to them.

People buy from people

It is important to understand who you are and what service you can provide. People buy from people so you need to start building a clear picture of you, your business and what you can offer. This will help you connect with your new clients and give you a voice and a message which is clear and concise.

Remember when your marketing, your new client is not sitting there waiting for you to post, or pop through their letter-box. More often than not they don't have the time to stop and read what you offer. But they will stop if you 'speak directly to them'.

I find that the response I get from my audience is far richer when I have an element of personality in my message. Even this book is peppered with sarcasm and humor. You may or may not relate, but that's ok. Something has resonated with you, which is why you have got this far down the first section.

Build your Elevator pitch

How do you introduce yourself to someone new? Do you fumble over the list of things you do? "Good morning I am an international nail artist and educator, I am a nail technician & salon owner, education consultant for a well-known international brand, creative director, an international judge and feature writer, columnist and author,"………take a breath…." how do you do."

I think I lost you at 'I am a…'

I have many titles, and it's common for us to trip over our roles. But there is one thing I missed out. I am a businesswoman and the other roles pale into comparison. If I come in and introduce myself to you as a woman in business, you more likely to respond with "What line of business are you".

Does your introduction get attention or lose it?

Let me give you a couple of examples.

"Hi, My name is Sam and I am a Nail technician," -

What's your first impression? Slightly underwhelming - what do you get out of me being a nail tech - am I trying to 'sell you' my services?

Let try this one?

"My name is Sam Biddle, I have 2 global enterprises providing education, inspiration & products to nail professionals, I am also quite famous in my field,"

So how does that go down? What's your first impression? I am slightly overconfident, overcompensating, do you believe me and why should you? I have not given you any reason to trust me at all, in fact, I sound a little full of myself.

Your introduction is a Sales platform you CAN'T sell from, it is important that you create a sense of trust and intrigue right from the start.

Who am I to you?

You don't care who I am because you have no investment in me right now. Are you interested because I have distribution networks worldwide and develop my own products? Are you interested in my industry at all? Do you know I inspire men and women globally and I have an online network of students I mentor?

The answer is most likely No to all of those and why would you; I have not told you yet and if I have you have probably switched off because it doesn't relate to you.

I need to sell myself to you, to ensure I have you listen to what I have to say - I have to figure out and translate in my introduction something relatable to you. So let's not concentrate on who I am, but instead what do you want from me?

Once I can give you something right from the start, I have your attention.

You could call it Machiavellian or manipulation...

Learn the art of reading people's wants and needs and then giving it to them in your introduction. Before they know it they are hooked into what you offer them. So lets get started.

Who are you?

- What do your clients gain from knowing you?
- What do you offer your clients and how can they benefit from you?
- What will your clients learn from you?
- Do your clients relate to you?

REMEMBER; people will always think about what you can give them. So you must consider your clients and what they want from you, then think about how you should introduce your business to them.
Take a few minutes to write the answer to the above questions.

Why you need to change the way you approach your customer.

Sell yourself through education, by providing your new client with something of value for free. I promise you they will pay attention to the next thing you have to say. When you come into your client's life, your introduction should stimulate the need to want to know you and what you offer.
If you can master how to educate through an introduction, tell them something they didn't know about what they are interested in and be credible, you will then have jumped over the first hurdle.

A couple of points to consider when your selling, but not selling is;

Sell your business.

I don't mean stand there and tell them the cost and price of each service, but
actually sell it by example. Give something away for free, be ethical in your approach, invite investment in kind.

Sell your products & services without selling.

Solve a problem before your client even know's they have one and educate them on the benefit of the services, not on the service it's self.

Being in Business is not about you or what you sell...It is about your client and what they want.

When I started there was no Facebook, it was just the power of referrals and door knocking. It helped that I was on the high street, but I had to get creative with my promotions. Local radio shows, and leaflet dropping increased awareness locally. I also became very active in the community and supported all the local events with a small nail art booth for the kids.

When Facebook arrived I had no idea the power behind social media, (I think no one did really.) I got my voice out there at the start and gained momentum as the online nail community grew.

As a free form of advertisement, I used it to build my business and targeted other nail professionals, my business was education. Now I have to pay to get my voice heard through ads and pay per click so marketing my business has become more refined and complex in the last few years. With timelines full of adverts, the consumer is not so quick to click. SO, I have learned it is not just about the delivery - but the message as well.

It's important to create loyalty and following from the start with an attractive introduction to you and your business, Give and you shall receive, by providing them with free Education, you will give your clients a reason to buy into you.

What's in it for you?

Hey, I get it; I am about to ask you not to ask for the sale, to share a lot of information with clients for free, so why should you waste your time doing that?

- Your clients will learn to trust you.
- By investing in them, they will invest in you.
- You will create brand awareness & loyalty.
- They know where to come and get more information.
- Understanding what your customer wants and needs comes before your business methodology.

So now you know why let's get you started.

You need to create an elevator pitch and a brand ethos. Now I am not talking about pages and pages of words. This can be only a couple of lines. You need to sum up your business and what you offer, keeping in mind everything you've learned about what your customer is looking for.

An elevator pitch is a persuasive speech you used to spark interest in what you do. A good elevator pitch should last no longer than a short elevator ride of 20 to 30 seconds, hence the name.

You need to craft something which is interesting, memorable, and succinct. It should also explain what makes you and your services unique. If you understand who you are and what you do, you will become more relatable to your audience. Most of us know what we do, but do you know what you offer and how to deliver that message?

1. Identify your goal
Start by thinking about the aim of your pitch. For instance, do you want to tell potential clients about your salon? Do you have a great new service you want to sell? Or do you want a simple and engaging speech to explain what you do for a living?

2. Explain what you do
Start your pitch by describing what your salon does. Focus on the problems you solve and how you help people. Ask yourself this question as you write:

What do you want your audience to remember most about you?

Keep in mind that your pitch should excite you first; If you don't get excited about what you're saying, neither will your audience. Your pitch should bring a smile to your face and quicken your heartbeat. People may not remember everything you say, but they will probably remember your enthusiasm.

3. What's your unique selling points?
Your elevator pitch also needs to communicate your unique selling points or USP.
Identify what makes you or your idea unique and add this after you have explained what you do.

4. Engage with a question
After you communicate your USP, you need to engage your audience. To do this, ask an open-ended question

(questions you cannot answer with a "yes" or "no") to involve them in the conversation. You might ask "So, how often do you have your nails done?"

5. Put it all together
Put all the elements of your pitch together and read it aloud, use a stopwatch to time how long it takes. It should be no longer than 20-30 seconds. Otherwise, you risk losing the person's interest or monopolizing the conversation.

Edit out words or things that need not be there, the main aim is to incite interest, and they will come back to ask more if your elevator pitch has worked. Then you can add the other cool stuff you do. Remember, your pitch needs to be snappy and compelling, so the shorter it is, the better!

6. Practice
Marketing is not just advertising, it is how you present yourself and promote what you do. But if you stumble over your elevator pitch, then you won't install confidence, so practice makes perfect, If you don't practice, it's likely you'll talk too fast, sound unnatural or forget the important stuff in your pitch. You want it to sound like a smooth conversation, not an aggressive sales pitch.

For example, if I was targeting someone for my online course;

"Hi my name is Sam, I mentor nail professionals to build confidence in their art and develop and grow their businesses. How do you feel about nail art?"

Or if I was targeting someone for this book;
"Hi my name is Sam, I work in the beauty industry, helping professionals grow their profits with marketing strategies, how do you feel about social media and having to advertise online to get seen?"

So now it's your turn;
- Work out your USP
- Figure out who you are to your clients
- Write out your introduction, relating to the product you're promoting

In the next chapter, we will discuss audience's (clients) and how to target (find) them. (When I say target, I really mean sell to, but I promise there is no selling!)

Your Ideal Client.

Once you have established what you can offer, you need to build a profile of your perfect client. This seems so far removed from work and marketing, I know you're probably rolling your eyes and wondering where this is leading. Well, I certainly did when I first learned this trick. But trust me, it helps.

I have my "ideal student" building up a profile of her likes and dislikes means when I build my message it is like I am talking to her directly.

When I did this, I saw a big difference in my sales and the growth of my business.

Building your 'ideal audience' should only take a few minutes. Grab a sheet of paper, and write out a few words about who you think they are, here is a list of some things to help you come up with a profile.

- Who; who are they, how do you know them?
- What; what do they want when they come to you?
- When; when do they come into the salon, need a treatment or visit social media?
- Where; where do they live?
- Why; why do they like coming to you and not the competition?
- Gender; male, female or gender-neutral?
- Personality; bubbly, reserved, etc?
- Age; this is important, for the services you will offer?
- Family life; married, have children, single, divorced and dating, widow?
- Job title; corporate or creative?
- Job function; are their hands in water, do they work outside?
- Income; can they afford you?
- Needs; what do they need from you, haircut, pedicure, nail art?
- Pain points; what do they want to change, what don't they like?
- Challenges; what do they find difficult, money, choosing colours, etc?

I have given you some suggestions, but build a picture of each one of your clients. You don't have a one size fits all, you will have 3 or 4 'types' of clients, for example, you might have;

Mary Jones who is 50 years old and retired. She loves working in her garden. Her children have left home, and she is expecting her first grandchild. She and her husband go on three holidays a year and have a good income. She is lively and loves wearing bright colours.

Jenny Smith works in a bank. Divorced but not dating. She has 2 young children and not a lot of money. She likes to play netball and plays for her county team. She is always on the go and doesn't spend much time pampering herself.

Sandra Robinson is a self-employed woman in her early 40s. Her children are both at university and she runs a small candle-making company, she likes to look good and is always wearing makeup and on time. She is divorced but dating and enjoys weekend city breaks. She drives an Audi convertible and loves being the centre of attention.

 So now I have three profiles It gives you a clue to where to look for them, and what to say when you find them. The trick is to change the words on your post, and what you're promoting to resonate with each of your ideal clients and their likes and dislikes.

I would not direct my special offer for a moisturising manicure for gardening hands and how to maintain skin when you're toiling soil to Jenny, she is not interested in gardening and doesn't have the time or money for a deluxe manicure and pedicure. You would direct that offer to Mary who can afford it and spend at least a couple of hours in the salon. Instead, I would target other treatments like hair or massages to Jenny. Sandra would have a lot of the additional luxuries, the things that set her apart from her peers. Hair extensions, Botox, nail art or non-surgical facelifts. Sandra has an image to maintain, so I would speak about these things when targeting her.

So I know what I need to push to each of my customers, but where do I find them?

 Will Mary be on Facebook? Highly unlikely, instead I would promote the gardening package in free local magazines and papers. I would leave my flyers and leaflets at garden centres. I would not waste valuable advertising space on the luxuries or the bargain basement deals and aim my conversation at the midpoint of the market.

Can you see where I am going with this? I can provide you with a list of places your clients might hide but until you can recognise them it is pointless going there.

Work out what you provide, what they want and make a small profile for each package.

You will have many clients with various needs and wallet size. So it is important to target them appropriately. But if you don't have any clients, then you can make up your ideal client.
Mary is perfect and Sandra will spend money with you. But Jenny is a hard sell, think about what type of client your looking for, and create the perfect profile.

Now I'm going to be honest with you, I found this hard to do because it felt like I was making it all up. It was only when I thought about them as characters of a book, and then drew inspiration from people I knew around me, that it became easier. My mother, my neighbour, the lady behind the supermarket checkout. Then I was able to form my ideal 'cleint profiles."

Help your clients to find you.

Where are your clients hiding? We have worked out who they are, but now we need to find them- It's like a game of hide and seek, but when you find them, you can't just tag them and run. There is more work to do.

This book is concentrating on social media as this is everyone's primary focus, but it's important to point out something vital. What would you do if there were no social media? I had to dig deep into my memory banks and remember the days before Facebook. What did I offer my clients to entice them into my salon and keep them coming back for more?

So I think we should start there because I see all too often social media marketeers become lazy with their approach to advertising themselves. Your social marketing strategy should be part of the bigger picture.

I assume that most of you reading this book are salon based or offer services in one area. This makes life a lot easier.

Online groups are a good starting point for targeting locals, like community groups, neighbourhood watch or buy, sell and swap groups. But it's important that this is not the only place you promote. Be visible outside of social media and away from the phone or laptop. You need to make sure that your clients can connect with you; I found the best way to do that is with a leaflet drop.

Arghhhhhhh! I hear you, it's costly, time-consuming and takes a while to get a return. I know, but can you imagine reinforcing your message on their timeline with something popping through the door the next morning?

There are three key things to remember with any marketing strategy;

1. Consistency - keep everything the same and make sure you do something at least seven times before you can expect a return. This includes a leaflet drop with the same message or posts with the same promotion. Your logo needs to be clear and recognisable.

2. Three-pronged attack - you need to come in on three sides, social media, through their letterbox and if they have signed up to your newsletter through their inbox. (We will discuss this more in a later chapter.)

3. Referrals and word of mouth. This one is hard if you're starting out, but solvable. Visit local shops around your salon or in the local area and offer your service out for free in exchange for referrals and recommendations. If your salon is in a small parade or local to someone who has a high social standing, offer them some free nail art, a hair colour or even a massage. Which they can show off and get complimented on or talk about. Make it clear that this is an exchange, you expect recommendations and referrals for the free treatment. If you're established but want to grow, use your existing customers and incentivize referrals. Get them to bring in a few friends in exchange for free treatments or a gift.

Trust me, the investment you make in doing the free service will pay off.

We have established the bigger picture when it comes to marketing and the fact it is not all online, so now it's time to put the cherry on top of our marketing sundae.

Let me explain, meet Margaret. You have not met her yet; she is a mother of 2 boisterous boys aged 7 and 9.

She has received your flyer through the door but not read it, recognising the bright pink heading and vibrant logo as a salon, she pops it on the fridge- maybe she will find time to pamper herself someday. She has heard about you, her neighbour, Sarah, had a wedding to go to and she had nail art painted on her toes and her hair put up. Margaret was mildly jealous as Sarah showed off her nails and raved about you and your new salon.

Margaret and Sarah also chatted about how terrible it was that the council were shutting down the local play park due to lack of funds. Margaret is feeling frustrated because she let's the boys play at the park right across from her house and she enjoy's a little alone time.

Now they are stuck in her garden running in and out of the house every five minutes. There is talk about keeping it open but they needed to raise the funds.

The next day, Margaret is on social media and reading in the local online group about the charity trying to keep the park open and how she could donate. Thinking she will donate later when she gets home, anything to help keep that park open, she thinks.

She scrolls on, the next post is yours, your bright vibrant logo, helping her recognise you. The large letters on the post say SAVE OUR PARK one manicure at a time. 'Strange' she thinks, she clicks on the post and reads about your special offer. How with every mani and pedi bundle booked before the end of the month, the salon will donate £5 towards the charity.

Can you see where this is leading?

You have targeted Margaret, by understanding the local community and attracting her attention with an incentive offer. She can kill two birds with one stone, support the charity and get the manicure and pedicure she's always wanted. She has a good impression of you, your professional leaflets, the recommendation and now your support of something Margaret also finds important. You have made a client for life!

You see with all the marketing you're doing offline, those clients are seeing your name and logo whilst hearing about you in conversations even when they pick up your leaflet to put it in the bin, (remember those flyers through the door the first 6 are likely to find a home in the bin, but they are still making their mark, even if it is subconscious.)

All this work, even if there is no immediate return means your new client already feels like they know you, the subliminal message and visual cues are doing the trick.

Let's change the end to this story a little to enforce the argument.

We know Margaret feels upset about the park closure and is reading about this on her Facebook group; she scrolls on and see's a photo of a set of nails, no words, no link to the website or even a shop name. She doesn't even recognise or relate, having no interest at that moment in nails. She has not been teased, tempted or given the opportunity to ponder on getting a manicure from you, so seeing a random set of nails in a group, is just that, random. Facebook will soon kick it out and no one will see it at all.

We have talked briefly about the power of marketing as a whole, but yes social media will probably be your main source of promotion. The best thing to do is figure out which platform your clients are on. If they are younger (30) and below you might find Instagram more popular. But don't rule out Facebook. Fast becoming an information platform, it is also a good way to offer your services.

There is one thing to always remember- your clients are not on social media looking for you. When your post pops up in front of them it must add value. The last thing you should do is sell. Facebook (and every other social media platform) wants to show users content that is most engaging and will drop everything else. What does this mean? Well, if your post is not getting the views, likes and comments, Facebook will deem this as not engaging and will not show it to your friends and followers. Death to your social media marketing in other words.

Focus your efforts on the right places

Don't waste your energy on multiple platforms. With Twitter, Pinterest, Instagram, Snapchat, Facebook, Linkedin, Google etc, you might think you need to be present on them all. But this will dilute your time and efforts so pick one as your main and focus on that.
To choose the best platform is to choose the one your audience hangs out on, it's that simple. Just because you don't like Instagram or understand it, doesn't mean you shouldn't learn. Most of your clients might not have your hang-ups and you could lose out on a lot of followers. Look for your competitors, where are others in your industry posting? If you don't see them anywhere on the platform, odds are you shouldn't be there either.

Optimize your social media profiles

We will discuss this more in a later chapter, but it's important that every aspect of your social media profile works for you. Your username should be easy to remember and relates to you. No z at the end of a word or using numbers. If someone is searching for 'Nails by Sam', that is what they will type in. They might not remember or know that you have spelled nails like this; 'N8ilz'.
Your logo and photo must be clear and recognisable, people need to become familiar with you and what you look like.

Call to action

What do you want your clients to do when they see you online. Will you be asking them for their email address to sign up for a newsletter or promoting your salon website? Whatever you do, you need a 'call to action' this is something you're asking your followers to do. Otherwise what's the point of posting. Promoting yourself goes so far, but if someone can't find you or connect with the minimal effort, then they will scroll on.

Post or promote?

There is a balance to posting. You don't want to sell sell sell your services in every post. It seems desperate and it will turn people off. They will not engage, like or share. But if you post content which people like- a gif, positive comment, happy or funny meme or helpful hint or tip, then you will engage your clients and get them thinking and sharing.

Then you can throw in the odd little promotional post. If your posting in a group, NEVER promote. It's like walking into someone's home and trying to sell them some handmade jewellerywithout an invitation. Use posts to promote and create an awareness of what you are, but don't sell. You can hint to your business and if people want to know more, they will follow through by clicking on your profile.

For example, posting on a group about something that's happening in your salon, or a top tip, will be more beneficial to a group and the admins will allow it. The hope is the followers in the group will hit the link and see your promotional posts on your page. I shall cover posting in depth in the next chapter.

Work smarter, not harder

Facebook has said the average user is subjected to over 1,500 stories per day.
So posting more is not the answer, posting 16 times a day will not increase your social presence instead focus on posting high-quality, relevant content.

Quality over quantity, posting less often will increase organic reach, and will save you a bunch of time, spamming your page 8 times a day with anything you can find is not good practice.

Posting once or twice a day should be enough, experiment with the timings and where you post. This is a guideline, you might find once a day or even three times a week enough.

Also, posting times make a difference too, most people wait and post when everyone is online, but really that will just throw your stuff in the middle of a big pile of posts hitting Facebook or Instagram at the same time. Posting during slow hours pays off and stops your post from drowning in the noise online.
I suppose I have taken it for granted that you understand what organic reach and paid reach means, and that the words and blurb you use in a post is what I mean when I say content. But in case you don't, we do cover this in more detail later in the book.

Engage your audience

Social media is a two-way street. It's not just a platform for businesses to promote themselves. It's a place to engage and interact with real people to create genuine connections for your brand.

Respond to the people commenting on your content, for example, if someone says "I want this!" on a photo of your product you need to reply with "So glad you like it! If you're interested, grab your own here!" with a link to your website.

People will look for your posts because they'll be genuinely interested in what you're doing. Forging a bond and responding to them is vital, especially in our type of business.

Responding to their comments and giving them help goes a long way to building customer loyalty, but is also helped by word of mouth. The more interaction you can gain, the more impressed someone is. They will definitely be talking about you.

Nurturing your clients.

Catching your clients and keeping them can be tricky. A client chooses you for many reasons, you would like to think it is your excellent work, but if I'm honest, it is probably more a case you're either the best value or closest. They will, however, stay with you because of your work and how they feel about you over a period of time.

We have already established the philosophy of 'build it and they will come' does not work regarding salons, mainly because there is a lot of competition. Learning your craft, attending workshops and then hoping and praying your clients will find you will just not happen.

How can you expect your potential clients to know what you can do for them if you don't tell them? But even if you tell them, they are actually only interested in 3 things.

This is the reality of the situation, the 3 things your clients decide on when they choose you;
1.   **Cost**
2.   **Distance**
3.   **Quality**

Sadly, in that order. But don't worry, you need not roll out a rock bottom price list and undercut the competition. In fact, this would be a big mistake, because you will always struggle with a small profit margin.

Instead, you want to tell them why they should choose you, what value you bring to them and how their choice will deliver something they couldn't get elsewhere or even dream to expect from the competition.

I am not talking about over-promising either; it is a simple case of reverse psychology.

Understanding why your clients book a treatment is the secret to getting a full appointment book. For example the three main reasons your clients think about having their nails done are;

> 1. FOMO; fear of missing out. They see others with beautifully manicured nails and think "I want some of that!"
> 2. They are not happy with other parts of themselves and feel nails, just like a haircut helps their self-esteem
> 3. They want something they don't have. Looking at badly bitten nails and wishing for long elegant talons is a great incentive to book an appointment.

So give your clients an ideal scenario, a perfect finish or immaculate ending to the vision and then present them with the reason you can give it to them all within budget, and little time.

Understanding this psychology means you can be proactive with your marketing.

Giving a solution to a pain point is an easy way to promote your services, on Facebook, with a mail drop or if you're lucky enough to have a mailing list- with a quick email.

How do you keep those clients sweet?

Just because you have a full appointment book and regulars, does not mean you can afford to be complacent.

There are a few simple tricks you can do to delight your clients when they walk through the door, open their mail after a long day at work or read a post on Facebook. You see sometimes your work is just not enough and you need to dazzle a little honey from time to time to keep them loyal.

Tiny trinkets to say "thanks" and "we love you" gifts is a sure-fire way to bring out a smile on even the biggest sourpuss.

A physical gift goes a long way and need not cost a fortune. There are many online shops, discount stores, and bargains to be had. Sometimes you don't even need to spend a penny, there are many companies and brands willing to send you freebies and samples for your clients to try.

Giving away a free nail file to my clients would be like I had given them a winning lottery ticket. A small bottle of hand moisturiser in their bag as they are walking out of the door or a hand full of sample sachets is like giving candy to a baby.

Turn a frown upside down when you bring them their coffee and a mini cupcake in a take-home bag for later. Buy your clients a coffee, literally! Give your clients a voucher from the local coffee shop for a free coffee, it might not even cost you a bean (a coffee bean, see what I did there). You see having an affiliation with other local businesses means a free little something for a client and a new customer for the coffee shop, a win-win situation for everyone.

There are many creative ways to keep your clients sweet, something as simple as a hand-written card in the post to say thank you for being an awesome is enough.

A little effort goes a long way, and it's not an every month thing, twice a year is enough to have a chorus of clients singing your praises.

Drowning a Complaint with Sam's secret sauce.

It might be a little early to talk about complaints here, but I really thought it would be helpful. Marketing is all-encompassing and not just about promotions and advertisements.

How you talk to your customer's and deal with their frustrations will help you gain new customers. Hear me out here!

So you're on Facebook and you see a post pop up of a text conversation which is getting rather heated and out of hand. Ending in both parties being rude.

This is a conversation between a client and a salon owner… eeeeek!

1. This should never have been discussed on Facebook and
2. That conversation should never have gotten out of control.

Any rejection you receive hurts because what you do for your clients is to the very best of your abilities and you would never set out to harm or con someone out of their hard earned cash with avshady service. So when they come at you and say "hey my nail fell off" YOU HEAR "You're a rubbish nail tech and your work sucks."

It's vital we stop at the moment we receive any complaint or critique and think about the words you're hearing and forget the emotional response it brings up.

Yep, basically, that means don't take it personally.

There are always two sides to every story, and when someone says something, it's coming from their experience. In reality, they don't give two hoots about you.

So how do you get over the sense of rejection? That is simple... take a breath and imagine yourself in the shoes of the person coming to you. If she seems a little cross or upset, well there are probably three reasons for that;

1. She has built up this confrontation in her mind to such a degree she is already expecting your response and is ready for a fight; it is a case of kill or be killed.
2. She is genuinely upset but does not blame you, just wishes it hadn't happened, your reaction to her frustration will either dismiss her feeling's or edify them.
3. She is a total bitch and out for a refund, regardless.

So how do you go about appeasing a customer and keeping them sweet? Well, it all comes down to honey, you need to drown them in it. In the nicest possible way of course!

1. Always put yourself in their shoes, think about the situation as if it was happening to you.
2. Never be defensive and never suggest you're right and they are wrong. Although this might be the case, it is sometimes better for the outcome to take the high road. If you do, deep down your client will know the truth.
3. Never suggest a reason as to why something happened or an excuse. Do this AFTER you have apeased your client, and the situation is in resolution.

So, let's put practical examples to those suggestions...

Mrs Biggs comes in, slams her hand on the desk in front of you and your client and says "My gems have fallen off!"

Here are two scenarios...

WHAT YOU WANT TO DO;

"Excuse me, I am with a client, I can't speak to you until later and there is no need to shout at me, I will sort this out,"

WHAT YOU SHOULD DO;

"Oh, my gosh Mrs. Biggs, that is definitely not good. I want to fix that for you right away, I am with this client at the moment but can I arrange a time you can come back and we can sort this out for you?"

Yes she was rude, Yes you were in your rights to reprimand her behavior, but do you think it got you anywhere?

The second option validated her dissatisfaction, and your calm approach with an instant solution meant there was nothing more to say. It also shows the client you're working on that you treat every client's nails like they were your own and understand if they are not happy, you will do something about it.

You need to be the bigger person here. You're in business and part of that means you have to manage people, including your clients. Think of it like being a parent, you need to have empathy, forget about pride and throw being defensive out of the door. There is something to be said about a calm, gentle approach, with open honesty and truth.

Have you heard of the Aesop's fable about the wind and the sun?

 The North Wind boasted of great strength. The Sun argued that there was a great power in gentleness.

"We shall have a contest," said the Sun. Far below, a man travelled a winding road. He was wearing a warm winter coat. "As a test of strength," said the Sun, "Let us see which of us can take the coat off of that man."
"It will be simple for me to force him to remove his coat," bragged the Wind.
The Wind blew so hard; the birds clung to the trees. It filled the world with dust and leaves. But the harder the wind blew down the road, the tighter the shivering man clung to his coat. Then, the Sun came out from behind a cloud. Sun warmed the air and the frosty ground. The man on the road unbuttoned his coat. The sun grew slowly brighter and brighter. Soon the man felt so hot, he took off his coat and sat down in a shady spot.
"How did you do that?" said the Wind.
"It was easy," said the Sun, "I lit the day. Through gentleness, I got my way."
I know what you're saying, but what if she demands her money back?

You will never change someone's mind if they go in asking for a full refund, they have worked their way into a frenzy and they feel, rightly or wrongly it is a justified request. The ONLY way to change this is to offer them something else in return.

Turn this negative situation into a win for both of you and make sure this client stays loyal to you always and validates your business with this one simple action.

If they demand a refund, ask them if they feel a full refund is an acceptable compromise for damage. Agree with them that you yourself would not like this to happen, so would prefer to rectify the issue immediately and as a gesture of goodwill offer a voucher of £5 off the next treatment.

THEN, and this is the secret sauce to keep that client sweet, post them a card the same day, a little something in the post is unbeatable, it shows them you're thinking about them and value them. In the card, thank them for understanding and allowing you to fix the problem. If you feel like it, throw in an additional sweetener of say a free nail art or gems or some kind of upsell on their next appointment.

How do you feel about all this? I bet you're thinking, that is a rather large amount of work for one tiny little break or a lost gem, but wait, think of this as a marketing strategy, this client will not only think you care but will also feel special and why not, she is special. It should make every client you have to feel like they're your only one. But as a marketing strategy, these ripples will travel far.

FB V's Insta

This is the one question I think I get asked the most, what is the difference between Facebook and Instagram and which one should I use?

You really need to understand the individual purpose of each social media platform and what its users want before you promote your self on there, it's also vital to appreciate the difference between them and not use the 'one size fits all' philosophy.

Instagram = visual platform, an image first, conversation second.
Facebook = network & connect, conversation first then the image.

Ok so maybe I have simplified it slightly, but I am trying to show you that there is a massive difference between these two platforms and therefore your approach should be different too. You don't want to be that person who hash-tags too much on Facebook or auto posts exactly the same message across both platforms at the same time.

There are many who think social media literally means social and you need to post, post, post as much as possible. Instagram and Facebook are each unique and are used differently.

The first difference that jumps out is that Instagram has younger users, with most Instagram users being under 30.

An advantage of being a popular social network for older consumers is that Facebook users have higher incomes. Understanding the age group of your followers and where they are likely to hide, should influence what you post where and how to adjust your message to make it more appealing to these audiences.

Facebook

The whole point of Facebook is to connect and build online communities. Pushing groups and communal spaces, Facebook is great for link sharing, new content, engagement and live video's. It means you can connect with different demographics and promote events worldwide should you need to. Another plus is their advertising platform, which I will talk about in more detail later on. One thing which works well is Facebook's ability to provide information to your new clients, through your business page and a detailed bio. You can also create an internal shop front, which could substitute a website, but I would not recommend this, more about that later in the 'turn a like into a lead chapter.'

According to the statistic's portal, in 2017 the average consumer spends over 2 hours a day on Facebook, so it still exceeds any other social media platform for users.

All this is just grand, but when would you use Facebook for your business instead of Instagram? Good question and one I will answer once you know just what `Instagram can offer you.

Instagram

Instagram is all about capturing moments and users interact with you in a very different way than they do on Facebook. You're more likely to find images which spark a conversation on this platform. Instagram users want to see authentic moments from your life, work or interests and are not looking at your business information or doing research on you.

Your followers have limited ways to interact with you, a comment or a heart is the only thing distracting them from scrolling on. Engagement appears to be far higher through Instagram. Perhaps the limited ways make it easier for those cruising social media.

Instagram is all about the hashtags where Facebook have a lower reach the more hashtags you use. Through Instagram, you can find and follow people based on the hashtags they use. Images are really what Instagram is all about and a picture tells a thousand words, the context of your post should be in that picture. If you can master that, you are halfway there.

There is an absence of noise on Instagram, a lack of distraction which allows you to scroll and enjoy the imagery and art.

You will not find games, ecards, memes or Kickstarter campaigns on Instagram and it leaves your timeline clean and clutter free.

You will find I talk more about marketing through Facebook in this book, and reference Instagram. That is because I find I get a better return through that forum. However, I get a bigger interaction through Instagram. I decided and would recommend that you do the same, choose one primary platform and stick with it. Don't be the jack of all trades and master of none. Instagram is my secondary platform, and I use it to share with my followers a 'behind the scenes" story.

If you don't have one yet...tsk tsk.

When Facebook started back in 2004, initially it was a networking platform for college kids; I'm sure you know the history of Mark Zuckerberg, but it was in in 2009 when it helped young professionals and brands to develop a voice over the internet.

Suddenly social media became a business tool and companies invested heavily into their social presence to attract fans and followers. Now companies large and small were all working on the same playing field, with advertising costs so low, it was now affordable to reach the masses through social media.

But if you're one of those like me, that started with a personal profile and nothing else, then a lot of your "friends" would be clients, students or other professionals.

It's time to upgrade to a business page.

Facebook wanted to separate the social from the business and has created a host of tools and benefits of creating a business page. Not only that if you continue to trade through your personal page, they could well come and take it all away, literally shut you down, and remove everything from your profile.

But don't panic, it's a good thing to have a business page. If you're using your personal Facebook profile to represent your business you're missing out.

But first, for those who just need to know, let me briefly explain the difference between the two.

Your Facebook profile

Plain and simple, a Facebook profile is a personal account on Facebook. When you sign up for Facebook, you make a profile. This is a place where you can add friends and family members, communicate on a personal level, share photos, videos, and life updates. Everyone who joins Facebook gets a profile and you can only ever have one under your name.

A Facebook page.

A Facebook page is a business account that represents your business, it allows you to promote to your followers who have "liked" it. Having a page also allows you to use Facebook advertisements plus there is no limit to the number of Pages you can manage.

Why should I have a business page?

Small businesses without a Facebook page can create the perception that your business is out of touch with technology and social media users. It can raise questions about the progression of your business and significantly hurt client trust.

Having a business page will allow you to build a following with no limitations. If you try to do this through your personal profile, then you will need to accept or send out a friend request first before connecting with a new client. In today's society people are not so happy to click accept if they don't know you. If you have a page, a relationship can start with a simple like.

Benefits of a business page.

I feel like I am selling you on business pages, but I have to stress, part of Facebook's terms are if you have a business you have to have a business page. So let me explain what the advantages will be for you.

Facebook Insights.

When using a personal page for business, you have no access to Facebook Insights. Insights help you view the metrics on your page's performance, learn which posts have the most engagement or views and also see data about your audience, including how to target them with advertisements.

Being able to track and measure results helps you improve your marketing and understand what is working and what is not. You don't apply your makeup without a mirror right? Well, make sure you can see what needs to go where when you're posting and advertising on Facebook.

Business Relevant Information.

When you use a personal page as a business, your business ends up with a gender and birthday. When you set up a business page, your business now has a category, a mission statement, products, awards, and reviews. If you want your customers to learn more about your company and what you do, you need to use this information

Direct targeting.

With a business page, you can choose your audience by country and age. This is great if you based in the Newcastle, England, you need not worry about people in Winnipeg, Canada trying to make an appointment with your salon.

Personal Profiles are Limited to 5,000 "Friends"

Even if you are a small business, plan and have the potential to grow your reach over 5,000 people on Facebook. But your personal profile is limited to that number, making growth impossible.

Personal Profiles look unprofessional.

Clients and customers are social media savvy now and used to seeing business page layouts and understand how to navigate them. When they click on your link and see a personal profile with your post about your fish and chip supper, mixed in with a luxury pedicure. You might miss the mark with consistency in your message.

Plus, your client would not be too pleased if she catches a post of you in the club, downing shots and looking wasted before her cut and colour the morning after the night before.

It looks sloppy and screams, "I don't know what I'm doing!" This is not the message you want to be sending out to current or potential customers.

Private matters

Most people set their privacy to reveal a lot of personal information to their "friends" on Facebook. As a business using a personal page, you're letting your customers read a personal insight to you, not only that, as your friend, they are opening their privacy up to the rest of your friend's list and it is not a safe practice in today's digital world.

Advertising advantages

This is one of those emotive subjects, "Why should I have to advertise?" There are many advantages to advertising and if you think about it, you can't expect the world to find you, you need to invest a little in your business to reach the audience you want, target those people with relevant interests and attract new fans and new customers. You can't advertise on a personal profile. I will talk more about advertising later on in the book.

So now you have established you need a business page, if you dont have one already, please put this book down and create one right away. Facebook have made it easy, but if you want to dig deeper and learn more about how to make the page work for you, you can join the waiting list for my new Marketing secrets online course here; https://sambiddle.co.uk/beinspired/sams-marketing-secrets-course-wait/

Can they find you?

So, now you know who you are, who you're targeting and what you need to say to keep them coming back it's time to tell the world. Well, Facebook anyway.

I know I have spoken about this already, but I want to push home the point to you again, It is vital you have a business page and DON'T (did you notice the bold capitals) use your Personal timeline for business affairs. Facebook doesn't like it, and they will punish you by removing everything off your account including you. It is heartbreaking to lose years and years of content in one hit, so your best bet is to move over to a Business page.

I am not going into how to set this up, as there are plenty of video's and courses out there to help you, but I want to give you 3 things to optimise your presence on that page.

There is a couple of places where you can improve your profile to say more about you. You'll be able to see in your insights just how many people click on your banner and profile image.

Do you have got something for them to read about your business?

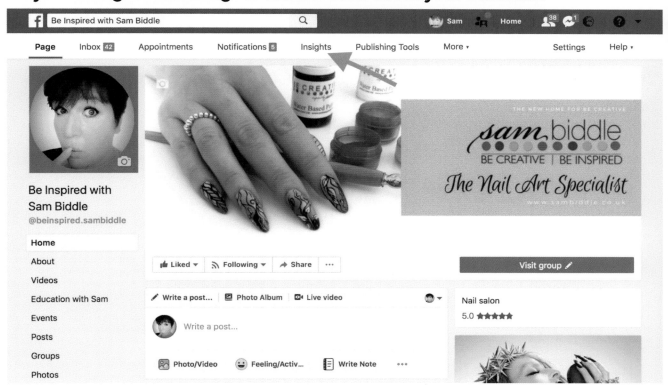

Banner image & profile image can do so much more for you.

All you need to do is make sure each image which reflects your business has a call to action, which is basically an instruction to the reader to do something like - book an appointment or call you. You can also use your elevator pitch here, to give your 'new client' more information about you too. If you have any offers or discounts, again, this is a great place to include them.

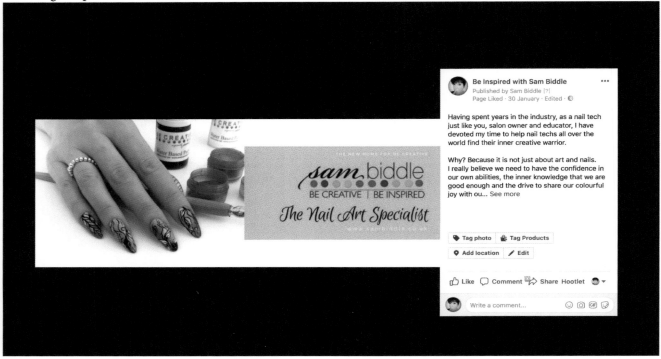

Your personal profile needs to send clients to your busines page.

Make sure your contact information is up to date and available under the ABOUT tab on your Personal page so it's a simple click for a potential client to find your salon business page.
 If you're working under your actual name, then it is likely that clients might look you up through a search on Facebook. If your personal profile pops up, then they should easily be able to find a link to your business page. I

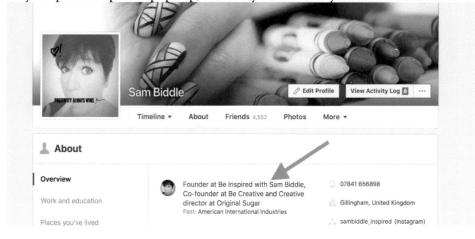

have taken a quick screenshot for you of mine. You can see there are a few pages to choose from. You need to link your business page in your "works at" section for this to show up.

When a Selfie works

It's important to use your face in your profile pictures, and not a group photo or an image of nails, pets or a building. People buy from people, they also will recognise you easily with an up-to-date headshot. So grab your phone and take a selfie and update your profile images today.

I would also keep the headshots the same across both pages, to keep continuity and help people find you. Having an image of your work for the banner across the top of your business page is perfect. To create a good banner image, check out Canva.com, it is a free editing app, and has great Facebook templates to help you build the perfect banner.

Below is my profile headshot, you can see there is also content in the post and a call to action, linking someone

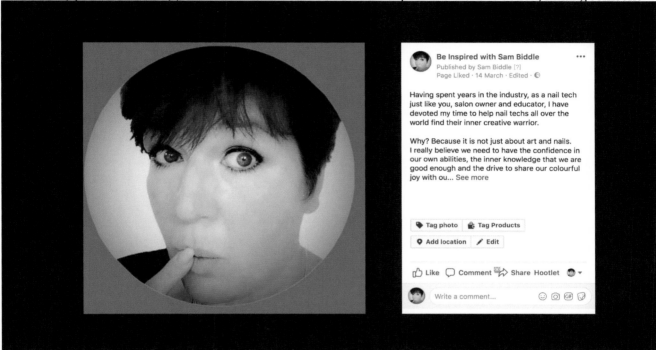

to my website and it also includes an email address.

You could have a call to action to subscribe to a newsletter or book an appointment too.

Add a call to action.

One of the main things you must remember is to tell your clients what you want them to do. Whenever you have a post, make sure you say "click my link to…" or "hit the blue button to message me" you can even use "book your appointment now by calling…"

It seems super simple, but it moves the client into an action.

One great thing about the Facebook page for your business is to direct your social media traffic onto your website or to sign them up to a mailing list. Facebook is a fabulous starting point to find your clients, but Facebook owns all your fans and followers. Without Facebook how would you access them? So make sure they know how to find you without Facebook. You also need to consider gathering email addresses from your clients, so you can target them in their in-box as part of the three-pronged attack.

Facebook also gives you an option to promote a website, your group or even a sign up list. With a big, blue button anchored to the top of your page, you can name this to ask your clients to do anything you want. From visit my website to message me. To change this, all you need is a link to where your sending your followers, click on the button and edit it to suit.

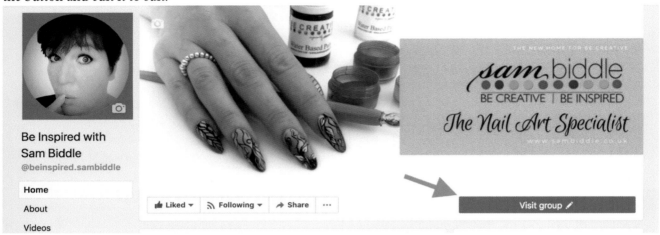

There is so much more to developing your business page and alot of different things you can do to make them work for you. This book is a guide to marketing and not a step by step instuction book for facebook. As much as I want to share all of it's secrets, I have to be mindful why you bought this book. I am developing an online course, to dig deeper into these things, you can join the waiting list here; https://sambiddle.co.uk/beinspired/sams-marketing-secrets-course-wait/

What to post where.

Not everything needs to be shared everywhere. This means not all content is suitable for every social media platform.

It's perfectly ok to create a post with entirely different messages on different platforms whilst using the same image. In fact, it might even help boost your engagement.

But how do you decide what to post on each social media platform? The main issue we all have is coming up with creative, unique and thumb stopping posts. With limited time it can seem like a thankless task. But trust me it is worthwhile.

What to post on Facebook.

Mostly, your goal with any social media is to build your brand and sell your services. As a Facebook Page owner, you're always trying to get more likes, comments or shares. You are far more likely to do this if you keep in mind that your posts should be about serving and not about selling.

Examples of selling posts would be;
- Times of appointments /availability.
- List of services
- Discounts

Examples of serving;
- How-to guides: information your followers will enjoy, be interested in or find useful.
- Top tips
- Humour and entertainment.
- Behind the scenes.

Video's work

Facebook is all about the live's and videos. And although it is difficult to place yourself in front of the camera, consider a small video of the salon, perhaps a treatment in progress or some nail art. Speeded up films of hair colour being applied, and art on nails are always popular.
But make sure you upload your videos to Facebook directly. Shares through YouTube links and from other sites tend not to get the organic reach you want. Facebook would much rather people stayed on their platform and doesn't encourage their users to hop over to YouTube for their entertainment. Post the same video on youtube seperatly and instagram too.

You shouldn't assume that videos will work for you so use a varied mix of images, status updates, links, and videos you post, but also use tools like Facebook Insights to track your posts and see which types are performing best.
Post the right balance of promotional/useful content, this is tough, because you immediately want to promote your product or service on social media. But you can't always think about yourself with these things. Users expect to find content that's useful to them, so sharing things like how-to guides, articles, etc will help grow a user's trust in you. They come to know you as an authority in the industry and will, therefore, trust you when you recommend a product or service in the future.

How to guides could include;

- How to make your hair colour last longer.
- How to give yourself a pedicure in 5mins.
- How to exfoliate with the things in your kitchen cupboard.
- How to find the perfect hair stylist.

Think of the 80/20 rule and balance your posts, Eighty percent of your content should be useful and helpful, while 20% can promote your brand or its products. That eighty percent will bring new followers and build trust, they'll then see the twenty percent and buy into what you're selling.

Don't forget that this variety should also include a mixture of videos, images, and other engaging content types.

How Long is long enough?

You have unlimited character length with Facebook posts as opposed to what the user will see on Instagram. But posts with 100 characters or fewer do far better than those longer.
But don't take my word for it, experiment and see what works best for you. When I am selling an online course, the longer posts with bullet points do far better and get more clicks, than something which requires my customer to go to a website.
But when I am posting a 'nurturing' post or a 'serve' post, questions or one liner always get great engagement. This is in my experience and you should experiement yourself to see what fits best for your market.

Ask a Question.

Questions are a great way to stop that thumb action. For example, instead of saying

"NAIL ART NOW AVAILABLE AT BE INSPIRED."

You could incorporate a question and offer options, to avoid a yes/ no answer.

"How do you wear yours?"

We want to know how you like your nails this summer. Plain, French, bright or bold. These are our favourite nail art looks.

Everyone loves a list.

Lists work really well for giving context and invoking intrigue. Break down some of your key points in your Facebook post into a few quick bullet points. Type this up in a note or on a document so you can include the bullet points or use emoji's, for more impact.

Example;

Three reasons you should get a gel polish pedicure.

🖤 *Shorter Drying Time*

🖤 *They Last Longer*

🖤 *Intense Shine*

Add a quote from your content

Give context to your post or image with a cool quote, uplifting message or even feedback from a satisfied customer.

Include an emoji or two 🛎️📸🪄😊

Emojis in your post can increase likes by 50%, and comments and shares by 30%, so go on, I give you permission to emoji away.

What to post on Instagram.

Instagram has become a place where people post only the best photos (and videos) on their profile.
If you sell physical products, I would avoid posting just the product. Remember serve not sell. Place your product in various settings. This would work with candid Behind-the-scenes shots of your service in action. As long as you maintain the arty, high res look, people will find beauty behind the picture.
Photo's of people in the salon, or clients, perhaps using a product are also a good idea. But the main thing to remember is that the image must have context. There has to be a story behind it which intrigues someone enough to stop scrolling and read.

Auto Posting

Trying to create content for every social site available can be time-consuming especially when you have a million other things to do.

Could there be a way around this?

For example, what if you just posted on Instagram and then auto-post it directly to Facebook? Surely that would save you a heap of time and effort.

Instagram has a cross-posting option and although tempting it will get you a far lower reach. Tailoring your content with a voice that appeals to the audience on that particular platform is by far a better option than selecting the auto share option.

You are better off using the same image and re-posting it on Facebook with a different message. It is also wise to post at different time, in case the same audience is following you on both platforms. The last thing you want to do is bore them.

If you use the cross post option, you will need to link your account to your Facebook business page. You will find at the post option you can switch over and share or not share to Facebook.

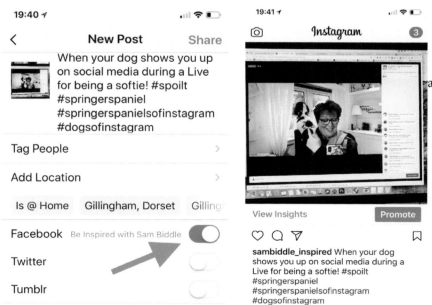

You only see 3 lines of texts on an instagram post, and will less characters available per post it is important to grab the users attention in the first line or two, to help add context to the image.

Use your caption on the image like a short blog post to share valuable educational content with your audience. Ideas of thngs you could post are;

Tutorials
You could share a tutorial on how to look after your cuticles or polish your nails. If you're a beauty therapist, you can share how to give yourself a hand massage. Make sure the image relates to the micro tutorial.

Tips and tricks
Bite-sized information on how to maintain your manicure or hints on how to extend the life of your hair colour.

Behind-the-scenes
Take your audience behind the scenes by using the caption to tell the story behind the image. For example, if you're sharing an image of a team member, you could expand on the story of their role in the salon.

Add Hashtags
Hashtags allow Instagrammers to discover content and new accounts to follow, we will cover hashtags in more depth later on in this book, I promise.

Encourage replies
Asking your followers to respond directly to your post is one of the best ways to increase engagement on your Instagram posts.

For example;

"I love red nail polish, what's your favourite nail colour?"

So now that we know the type of things to post and have delved into the knicker draw of these main social media platforms, lets discuss posts in more detail.

The low down on posts

This is it, probably the one chapter you will look back on time and time again and the main reason people have bought this book. What to post on Facebook and some tools and tricks to make your business page work for you.

Going Live

Facebook Live is a new and great way to interact and engage with your Facebook fans and followers. Lives will have a better chance of high organic reach and actually can be quite engaging.

But putting yourself in front of the camera, no matter how small is hard. What would you talk about? Perhaps a simple Q&A for your clients, getting the questions beforehand you can work through 3 or 4 during a live about manicure or hair colour. Depending on what your specialty is. Another great Live idea is a preview or unboxing of a new product, perhaps a colour swatch or a clients reaction to the smell of a lotion? One final idea is a behind the scenes look, perhaps a treatment or even an interview about a top tip to maintain hair colour. Social media is a window into your business, it doesn't always need to be perfectly polished. Creating content that takes your page visitors behind the scenes shows them what your brand is all about, helping to create a connection.

Eye-catching graphics

Facebook posts with images see over 200% more organic reach and engagement than those without an image. It's important to find a thumb stopping image to grab your followers attention and make them read what you offer.

Everyone loves a contest

Running a contest is one of the best ways to promote on Facebook. It's engaging for current followers and can help you reach people in your target market that don't know you yet.

One requirement to enter is to LIKE and share the post. This helps promote your contest to people outside of your network, increasing your chance to increase your audience.

Offers and discounts on your page

Offering special promotions on Facebook is a direct way to promote on Facebook. Creating an image with a 20% discount code word to use when booking before a certain date, works a treat. Make sure there is a call to action directing them to your online booking form or a telephone number to call.

Creating a limited-time discount jolts page followers into action. BUT a word of warning, Don't offer discounts all the time, as clients will just wait for the next one. Make sure you ask them to share the offer with their friends it might be something they rarely think about doing.

Educate

Educating your potential clients on the benefits of your services and the products you use. It will bridge the gap from awareness to desire. It creates a professional impression to your clients; you know what you're talking about and an authority in your craft. You're providing useful information relatable to them.

User-generated content

Featuring photos of happy clients, using your products or enjoying their beautiful new hair colour, reviews and thank you messages are a great way to generate third-party endorsement. It also gives a nice break from the polished and carefully thought out images and branded posts. People love people and will stop to read more. Giving your Facebook followers the spotlight is a great way to give back to your users while still promoting your product or service.

I had this campaign when my first book went on sale which had people posting images of themselves with my book. I did a call out for the most unique and original and continue to use them for my promotions.

This works because it creates social proof, acting much like a testimonial. Other potential customers see others like them, enjoying the product, so they feel like they might like it too.

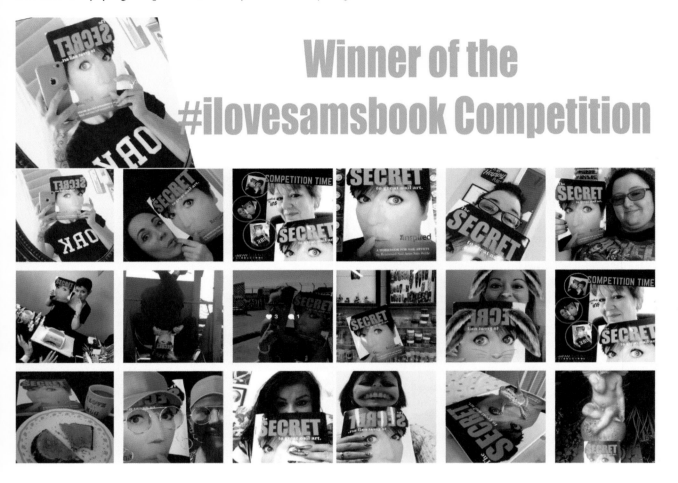

Capitalise on Trends

Posting about trending topics is one of the best ways to engage with your Facebook following. Creating content that reflects something in the media will resonate better with the people who see it. It shows that your business is in tune with what's going on in the world. Taking a step out of the promotional bubble many businesses get stuck in.

Make sure these trending topics relate to your industry, a release of a new Disney movie can lead to some great nail art examples online. Perhaps a treatment has been mentioned on a popular television programme, do you offer this? Refer to the programme and promote it. We have just had three different Winnie the Pooh movies released in the past 12 months, and although you may read this book in the future, we were certain to use this nail art in one of our posts, connecting it to the recent Christopher Robin movie.

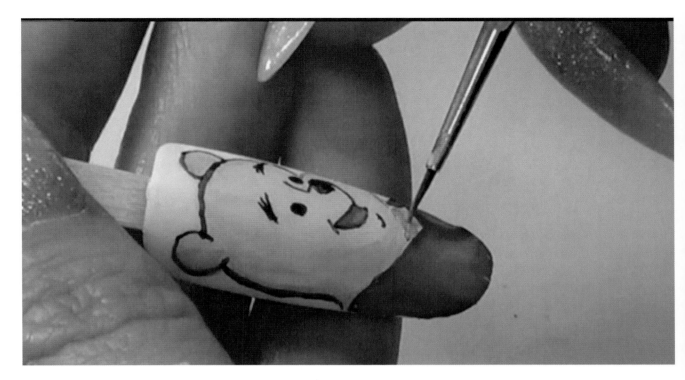

Pin a promotion

Another fantastic tool is to Pin your post. Facebook allows you to "pin" a post to the top of your page. Giving you maximum exposure for a campaign or promotion and making sure each visitor that checks your business profile sees it.

So now we have covered some of the types of posts you can use, you now need to understand the importance of structuring your post.

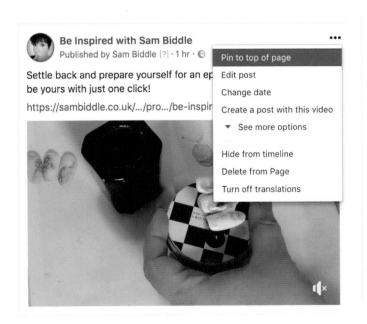

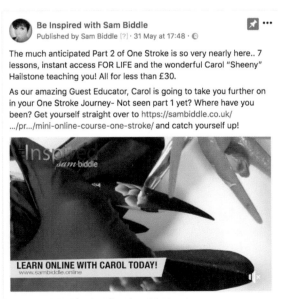

The power behind your post.

In this chapter I thought I would share with you my four-step process to posting on Facebook and Instagram. You should use this process in one post, but there are some important things to consider.
Remember, you your end goal, why are you posting, what do you need, more money, more clients, more likes? Also, don't think of posting as an individual process. Each post should be part of a bigger story or campaign. So every fourth post asks for the sale. The other three just serve.

Say this aloud;
Serve, serve, serve, Sell, Serve, Serve, Serve sell… and repeat

Also, make sure you're posting the right thing on the right page. Your business page is for BUSINESS, your personal page is just that, personal. Don't mix them up. You can see with this infographic what you should and shouldn't post on your business page.

  WHAT TO POST ON YOUR BUSINESS PAGE!

  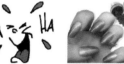 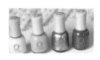

| A PROFOUND TRUTH - unless this is part of your brand keep it to your personal timeline | A COOL FACT - keep the subject nail or beauty related. a cool fact on how to get your kids up in the morning is not appropriate for your business | AN EMOTION - we all have them, if there is something which needs to be said then do this on your own time line. | FOOD - best posted on Instagram, avoid Facebook foodie pics at all costs on your business page. | A JOKE your brand is a reflection of you, your humour might not sit well with everyone, don't make them suffer your jokes. | NAILS & NAIL ART - an obvious one, but don't limit it to nail art, lip looks and beauty tips and tricks, you tube tutorials and get the whole look inspiration. | NEW COLOUR COLLECTION Don't forget to shout out about the hot new seasons colours now available a the salon. | SPECIAL OFFERS - keep this to a minimum, prices and offers only. You should be only have 1 a week and post this just once a day! |

Every post should contain these four elements;

Grab
Relate
Intrigue
Invite

Let me delve into each of them further for you, but jot down those four headers, and pop it on a post-it note, so the next time you fire up your laptop or desktop and schedule posts you will remember.

1. Grab Their Attention
You normally do this with a photo which should stop them in their tracks and be intrigued enough to read more.

2. Relate to their wants or needs

The image is not enough, to get a sale, I see all too often a quick post with just a film or an image, but no description, a call to action or explanation to attract the customer further into your story.

Below is an example of a simple post with a non-threatening call to action. You are not asking them to part with cash, you're inviting them into the salon. (Make sure you have the salon name and address under this), the nails

 Be Inspired with Sam Biddle

Published by Sam Biddle [?] · Just now · 🌐

Once or twice we need to add a little spice, a touch of danger and a bit of romance.

Sarah loved these nails, for her special anniversary dinner date. A perfect match to the outfit!

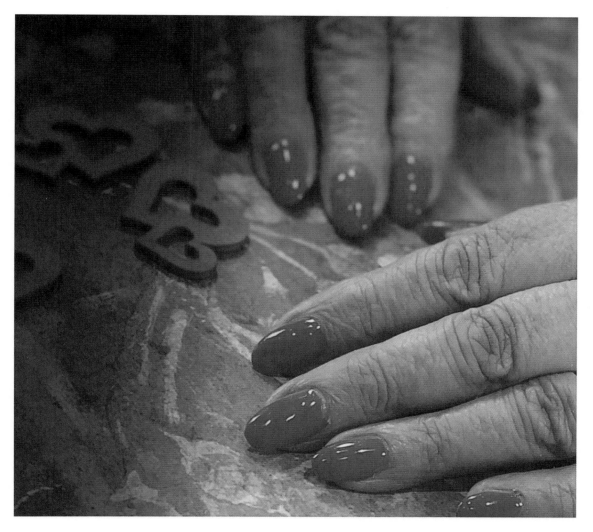

are plain, but the message might spark the imagination of the client.

3. Intrege

You want to peek their interest, but it's important not to sell. You should only ask for a sale or promote every third post. Check out these two examples, it is still a simple colour on a nail, but the background and props are makeing it complete and telling a story. Your words should also relate to the background and the nail colour.

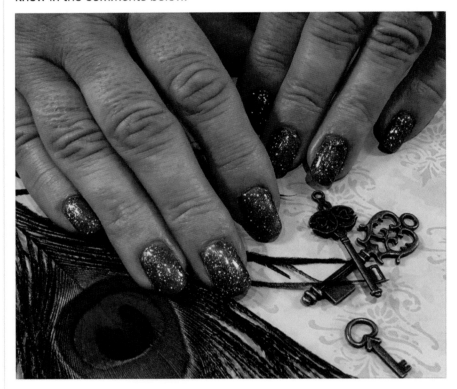

If you want to include props here are my top tips;

- A background that relates to what you're trying to say. Romantic, vintage, retro.
- 1 or 2 props max! The star of the show is the nails.
- Colour choice - keep it similar.
- Try to tell a story, or use the props as part of your post/message.

4. Invite and ask for the sale.

Like a good courtship, you need to woo and wow your customers! But then it's time to ask for the sale, it can be a simple promotion, a reminder you have availabilities or tell them you're looking for clients to have nail art. But there are major DON'TS for posting;

- Have post after post of just nails.
- Post after post of available booking slots, or cancellations.
- Complaints or rules.
- Lists of things you offer.

Remember this is Facebook, and those checking out your stuff are not looking for a bunch of sales, reminders or rules. They are looking to be entertained and amused.

This is an example of a good post, it is offering something, there is a call to action and an offer which might go away if they don't act fast. For anyone tempted to have nail art, this might be the push they need. Also, the nails are not over the top and easily worn for those afraid of art on thier nails.

 Be Inspired with Sam Biddle
Published by Sam Biddle [?] · Just now · ⊕   •••

Book your nail art today, and receive a FREE gift when you come for your appointment.

For the first 10 people, I have a special free gift for you. Bok today and we will tailor the art to suit your occasion.

Call me right now on 123456789

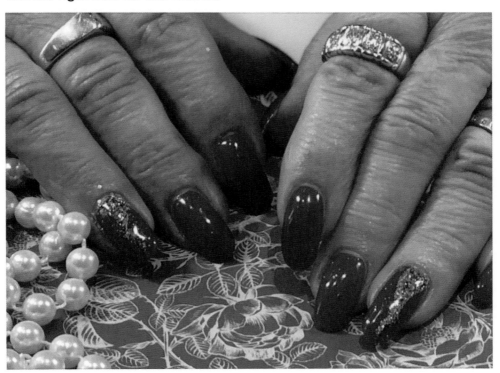

Hastags.

Once upon a time, the '#' was a simple symbol used before a set of numbers, but then its fairy godmother turned this mundane symbol into an online sensation.

You can find a Hashtag or two lurking on Twitter, Instagram, Facebook or any other social media post and there is no escaping them.

But what exactly is a Hashtag?

It's now one of those questions you're just too afraid to ask, for fear of looking and sounding social media illiterate.

And it's not just that "what" question, you're probably wondering why too. It will open a whole can of opinions and advice, but really you need to know the bare bones to make a Hashtag work for you.

If you're confused about Hashtags, join the group, I used to wonder what the heck they were for, but since everyone else was doing it, so should I. I asked my children since they seem to grasp the world of social media far better than me, but they made no sense at all. It was only when I was teaching a class in Sydney Australia that someone suggested I needed a Hashtag. One blank look later, It was explained when everyone uses that same Hashtag for my trip #SamBiddletakessydney and post their photo's on Instagram, Facebook or Twitter, one quick search later for that Hashtag and everyone's images come up in that search.

One massive lightbulb moment later and wow! Potential marketing opportunity, I got it!

So in a nutshell, Hashtags place your image or post amongst others of a similar theme or subject. So when people search for #roses then you will get a bunch of images from people who have posted about roses.

Hashtags have suddenly become a powerful tool to grow your social impact and engage your audience. Not bad from a lowly, hidden symbol on your keyboard.

So now you know the quick version of a Hashtag lets break it down a little further.

It's hard to make your images or posts stand out from the crowd, especially as we see thousands of them every minute across all platforms. If you use a Hashtag to index or mark your photo with a subject or theme, you will have a better chance for someone to discover it, even if those searching your theme or subject are not following you.

For example, you have just done a beautiful set of nails on Mary Jones and added a little pink rose to the corner of her ring finger, you could Hashtag #nailart #ringfingermanicure #rosenailart
Then someone who is not yet your client, searches for #nailart and boom, your beautiful pink rose mani pops up. She sees your local and you have a brand new client. Yes, it could really be that simple.

Why should you use Hashtags?

Because of Hashtags, your posts are no longer limited to just your followers. By adding one of these bad boys, your content will be accessible to all other users interested who search for that Hashtag.

Choosing the right Hashtag can expand your reach to thousands of potential new followers, fans or clients. BUT BEWARE if your hashtag is popular, like #nailart with over a million posts attached to it, the chances of being seen are as slim as I would love to be someday.

But if you add a specific tag like #Pinkrosenailart your post or image will have better odds.
There is a science behind Hashtags, and in your post, use three different types.

1. Content Hashtags
Use a Hashtag directly relating to your service or product if you're selling one. You can even include your industry or area of expertise. For example, I personally might use #nailarteducator. Or you could use #haircolourist, #nailartisit #beautytherapist.

A content Hashtags relates to the content of your content and will attract people who are looking for the things you're posting about. If you are posting nail polish swatches, then the Hashtags might be #nailpolishswatch. (I have just done that and there is over 122,546, however, those are better odds than the 15,876,022 associated with #nailpolish)

2. Trending Hashtag:
Another great way to boost your visibility is using existing Hashtags that are popular among millions of users, known as 'trending Hashtag'. But before you add the #, think, is your post going to add value or a different perspective to the topic, because if the answer is no then it will be ignored and lost, if yes it might be reposted by the millions following this trending #.
For example, if there is an emotive subject which gets a lot of attention like elections or even a royal wedding and you do nail art inspired by that subject, it's worth Hash tagging it. Perhaps you come up with a new treatment or service relating to a health issue which has a trending Hashtag then you would consider adding it. Even that nail art of Pooh Bear, in the last chapter, would get #christopherrobin #winniethepooh #winniethepoohnails

3. Brand-specific hash tags:
Using other more popular Hashtag might mean your post gets lost in the thousands of other people using the same tag, so consider creating your own brand-specific Hashtag. I have #inspiredonline and #sambiddle. You can also use one for specific promotions or events like I did with #sambiddletakessydney. On Instagram people can now follow Hashtags, so you can always encourage your clients to search for you on Instagram.

The key to creating an effective brand-specific Hashtag is to ensure that there is no one else using the same one. Make it unique and memorable by using a short motto or tagline. If you will use them in your marketing, you can give your clients a compelling incentive to use them.

For example, get users to post and add your Hashtag for a chance to win a free service or discounts.

How to use Hashtags wisely?
To create a Hashtag, all you need to do is include a '#' and the words needed to explain your post. This you should already know by now. But what you didn't know is that not all Hashtags are born equal.

1. Keep it short:
To save everyone the headache, don't squish too many words into one Hashtag. It was commonplace to Hashtag a sentence so your whole post became a string of words without spaces. Nothing turns people off more than lengthy Hashtags #Ineedcoffeefirsthtingeverymondaymorning.

2. Don't overuse:

Avoid (please, please) avoid writing your entire post with Hashtag in front of every word. #Because #this #is #super #irritating #to #read #and #makes #you #look #stupid! The general rule is to use a Hashtag next to words that are significant.

3. Think smart:

Use Hashtags which relate to your content, but are not overcrowded. I could add a Hashtag which is popular but then use one which is more specific as well.

How many Hashtags per post.

The more Hashtags you use, the more engagement you will enjoy but it seems anything over 10 Hashtags that engagement drops.

What's the best Hashtags to use?

This is where we need to be a detective, head over to your search bar and check out your competitors and other industry leaders. Pay attention to what they are using, the number of posts per week and how many Hashtags they add to their posts. Another thing to check is what their interaction is and the comments and hearts they get. You want to jot down the Hashtags to the popular posts. I add this into notes and copy and paste them into my Instagram post to save time.

Where to place your Hashtags?

Keep everything neat and tidy with your posts and I find consistency is key. It's best to put your Hashtags at the end of your caption preferably separated by either dots or asterisks. If you want to keep your post clear of the symbols, then you could add your Hashtags in a comment. (Ideal for those OCD and neat freaks amongst us).

Hashtags and Facebook

Believe it or not, Hashtags are not important on Facebook. Using the brand specific Hashtags or those relatable to the content can't hurt, but have only that. You should only really use 1 or 2 Hashtag's to make your post relevant or searchable. But some social media strategists say Hashtagging on Facebook can harm your organic reach so it's best to stay away.
Others say Hashtags can help your reach, the argument is still being debated, but the main rule of thumb is if you will not use Hashtags properly, then it's best not to use them at all with this social media giant.

Ask yourself, when was the last time you searched with a Hashtag on Facebook. To be honest, all you need to do is search the word and it's all there.

But if you want to post on Facebook and add a Hashtag or two, then here are three important things to remember.

- Keep your tags relevant. Don't add Hashtags which are popular but have no bearing on your post- that's called Spam and FB doesn't like it.
- Keep them short. Facebook is all about the conversation and when you clutter up the post with Hashtag symbols, it becomes less readable. Anything over 2 or 3 tags and you risk turning people off your post. (And Facebook too)
- Mix it up. Post a good mix of posts with and without Hashtags so when you DO tag with them they stand out more and make people take notice. I tend to click on a Hashtag if I haven't seen it before.

So there you have it, you are now an expert on hashtags, who knew there was so much to learn about this simple symbol.

Turn a like into a lead.

So we have a Facebook page, we have clients, we are in business!... But hang on a second, you and I know that clients are not always the same clients you started out with.
So how do we keep those clients coming back for more? Recommend your amazing services and the cherry on the sundae, adding onto their service which means more pennies in the bank for you.

So what do you do to get those clients to love you? Well, in plain and simple terms, you woo the pants off them; you nurture the relationship and watch it grow and develop into something wonderful. But if you're doing this through Facebook, then you're restricted to what Facebook allows your clients to see.

Facebook also owns these clients information, and we need to own them. If we can own them then, we can control what they see.
So you have a bunch of people who LIKE like your page, Now we need to convert them into a LEAD.

A LEAD is someone's contact information, they have allowed you to have their email address and said yes to receiving information via email through their inbox. This is a big deal because now, you can target them without Facebook censoring your information.
You will get a larger ROI (return on investment) through email marketing.

So how do we get those leads off Mark Zuckerberg and stop him from deciding what message gets seen by whom and when?

The first thing you need to do is sign up for a CRM service, there are many FREE email/newsletter CRM's out there, but I would recommend Mail Chimp at https://mailchimp.com. Sign up for a free account and build a list. It is super easy to use, with a ton of easy to follow instructional videos. This also makes it alot easier to deal with the new GDPR laws, and mail chimp will guide you with this.

So now you have a safe place to store these email addresses, you need to gather them. One of the quickest and most effective ways is to create a LEAD MAGNET - this is a free something or a discount your clients will get if they give you their email address.

Once you have their email address, then you can contact your clients drectly and not through Facebook. Basically you own those LEADS, and you can control when and what your client see's from you.
 But there is another really great advantage, you can target a post through Facebook to be seen by those on your list and their friends... how cool is that. So if you send an email out, about 'saving the park one manicure at a time" you can get facebook to post directly to those on your email list as well. Reinforcing the three prongued attack. So your client will not only see your email, they have a leaflet through the door, and when they next go online, they will see a post as well.

This is done by creating an 'audience' through facebook ad's mananger and then telling facebook that your post needs to be presented to those in that audience. If you have a website, you can even instruct facebook to collect everyone who visits your website into a list, and target them with a specific advert. This is going far deeper into facebook, and advertising, and something for the online course, which you can find more information about here; https://sambiddle.co.uk/beinspired/sams-marketing-secrets-course-wait/

Some lead magnet ideas could include articles on topics which interest your client, you can type this up and email them over as a reply with a thank you for subscribing email. You could offer them some free samples or bonus nail art when they come in with the printed email.

Other incentives could include;
- 3 step guide to a natural home pedicure.
- The trick to the perfect polish
- Free samples
- Bonus nail art with next booking
- Discount off a service exclusive to those on the list
- First to find out about new stuff

You can set up your Mail Chimp sign up from inside Facebook and gather those precious LEADS/emails addresses straight from your business page.

What do you do with your list?

So now you have an email list of clients who are interested in what you have to say and offer, you need to keep them interested. Don't just gather the list and leave it, or send out the odd - "I have a free appointment" announcement here and "buy this amazing product/service" there. That will turn them off super quick.

You want to think about the stuff you get in your in box, and what turns you on.... mostly that is the free stuff, right?

So instead of just using your mailing list when you feel like it, make a commitment and build a relationship with those clients.

As soon as they give you their email address you want to send out three fabulous emails which will have them hooked, full of educational information designed to serve not sell. Do this three times and in the fourth email, you can sell them something, give them an offer or ask them to do something, Like... share your Facebook page.

This is all automated through mail chimp, so it will happen while you sleep.
So let me give you an example of your emails.

EMAIL 1.

[SUBJECT LINE] now aren't you wonderful, you have just become my new best friend
[CONTENT]
Hi ..... add a name, mail chimp has a shortcut for this...

You are simply wonderful; I thought it was about time I told you that. It is always so lovely to be more in touch with people who love my page on Facebook and I appreciate you joining this exclusive little [.. add the name of your salon...] newsletter.

As promised here is your [give them a link to the lead magnet]

I will keep in touch with you and help you get the very best from your nail/ beauty/holistic/therapy/hair (add the one you want to focus on) treatments, you will also be the first to find out what's new, what's on trend and if there are any offers going on, because we all love an offer right?

As you signed up for this email, I will make sure you find out first.
So in the spirit of sharing, I wanted to share one of my big top tips that every client should know about.......[include something you can share with them, keep it short and sweet]

One last thing, could you do me a massive favour, and hit reply on this email, just so I know you got it ok, and if there is anything I can help you with, let me know in your email, otherwise a little 'yes I got your email' will do.

Now tomorrow I will send you something amazing, so check your inbox first thing, you will not want to miss this.
[end]

—————————————————————

Having them reply to the email, shows their email provider they want to receive emails from you, and your next email will hit their inbox and not get gobbled up by the frustrating spam box.

Mentioning the fact you have something else you want to give them 'tomorrow' sets you up nicely. They will be expecting an email from you and if your lucky, will want to read it.

EMAIL 2.

[SUBJECT] I told you-you would not want to miss this!
[[CONTENT]
Hello [insert name]

Yesterday you received an email from me with a big fat thank you, I am still super stoked you could join this newsletter list. Now I know what it is like getting a ton of emails about nothing much in your inbox, so I won't be sending you another email until later on in the month, but I promised you something super amazing in this one...

I wanted to thank you properly, yesterday I gave you my [lead magnet name], but I wanted to do more. Today as a special thank you I would love to give you an exclusive discount off your next pedicure. When you come in, whisper this secret code [insert code] and I will knock off...[insert amount]

Let me know if you have any questions, just hit reply to this email or message me on Facebook, here is the link;

[end]

—————————————————————

By giving them a discount code off their next treatment, or even a treatment they have not considered, you are inviting them back into the salon and expanding the goodwill. If you reluctant to give money off, consider this as a loss leader, the fortunes will come back to you when they rebook, but more importantly, they will be far more likly to open your next email. That is what you want.

EMAIL 3

SEND OUT 1 WEEK AFTER THE FIRST

[SUBJECT] So much has been happening at the salon, we are getting ready for...[insert holiday/ festival/time of year]

[CONTENT]

So [name]

I wanted to touch base with you, because we have been super busy in the salon getting ready for [insert holiday/ festival/time of year], but through with the power of technology you can find out all about it in the comfort of your own home with a coffee. So pop the kettle on and let me tell you...

[add what has been happening- you could include the following]
- New nail art designs.
- Achievement on a course.
- Discounts
- Client focus/testimonial/Facebook post - you can re-use stuff you posted

I hope we see you back in the salon soon, so I can show off all this, but I would also like to share something else with with you that I think you will find interesting…

[Insert top tip .... keep it short and sweet}

[end]

————————————————

The fourth email will be sales related, asking them for an action. Then you will revert to serving again in the 5,6 & 7t. Updating and maintaining your list keeping it warm.

It is really important that you don't bombard them with offers and turn them off, just butter them up, and slide a discount or offer over to them every third email. I promise you this will work.

So what else can you do with this list?

Build a relationship - For every reply you get, reply back, be their friend and thank them for their email. Again short and sweet.

Ask them to do stuff. - Send them back to Facebook and ask them to recommend and share your page

Recommendations. - This is always amazing once you have a personal relationship you will get more recommendations, but ask them to do a feedback testimonial post on FB for you.

So what should you NOT do with this list?

Don't let it go cold. - Don't ignore it, even if it is just once a month, send them something. Nurture your little seedlings and they will grow into beautiful flowers.

Give to receive - Don't just promote and sell, I know I've said it a few times but serving not selling will get you better results.

Never complain. - Please never moan or court sympathy. People do not want to put gold into a sinking ship, so make sure they know you're a good place to come.

Who's watching you?

This is going to be short and sweet, but I feel it is important to mention because I see this mistake being made time and time again. This is a friendly word of warning.

Drunk selfies and angry rants will not install a lot of confidence in your clients. Poor me posts will turn your clients off because no one will put their gold on a sinking ship.

Now you're in business, keep your business to yourself. Don't make it public. Even if it's on your personal timeline, please know people are watching.

Be professional all the time, and keep your personal and private life, well private.

Social media is now a tool to use for your business and not somewhere to vomit all your problems or show the world how wasted you can get on a weeknight.

This might seem a little harsh, but I want to shock you, especially before you shock poor old Mavis, when your antics the night before her blue rinse and set appointment, pops up on her timeline whilst she is eating her porridge.

Serve not sell.

When you hear the sentence "you have to sell" do you break out in a mild sweat, and quiver at the thought? SELLING gets a bad rap and it shouldn't. It's a beautiful thing, and if you're thinking, "Sam has lost her marbles" hear me out!

Selling is one of the most personal things in the entire world; it's two people saying "We both have a problem which we can solve."
For example, many of you who follow me, sign up to one of my online courses for nail art, buy Be Creative products or come to one of my face-to-face classes because you have a *problem*. You need to find an easier, better, more creative, more inspired solution to creating kick-ass nail art that your clients will love and buy.
I have a 'solution'- I have idea's, products, skills and techniques that will help you and I can share them with you.

BUT that's not where it ends... because I have a *problem*, too. And you have the 'solution' for my problem:
I need to feed my family, keep a roof over my head, and keep clothes on my back. This stuff isn't free. So I need money. In brief, we both have a problem, we both have a solution. Let's solve them by working together.

You have money to help me and better still, you can justify giving it to me because I'm giving something to you in return, my time, energy, expertise, and product or service.
It's an even exchange. I help you. You help me. We help each other.

I can solve my own *problem* of food/clothing/shelter by getting ANY job, there is nothing wrong with stacking shelves at Waitrose, I have done that!

However, that job was not the embodiment of the skills I've gained. It is not a way for me to share the gifts with you. It was not me being my best self and making the most of my talents and gifts.

You wanted to find out more about marketing your salon, and over the years I have gained a lot of knowledge in this area. It is a win-win situation for both of us.

That is the key to being OK with selling.
Don't be afraid to sell and never hide the fact you're doing it to earn money. I want you to be successful in your salon and business and with every word I type I give you all my secrets to being a success. In exchange I will earn a small percentage of the sale of this book, in order for me to continue to stay in business and help others. Using the serve not sell philosophy in selling, might just help you overcome your hesitancy. You're providing a valuable service someone is looking for and getting paid for it.

You have to pay to play.

Sadly, in this day and age you have to pay to play in the world of social media advertising. Facebook and Instagram have their own business model and advertising is part of that. I am going to, hopefully, guide you through the whys and wherefores in this section of the book, and make it as painless as possible.

But one thing is a certainty, this form of advertising is probably one the cheapest (except word of mouth) and effective. If you imagine being able to have access to the right people at the right time for just a fiver and let them know about you, it is a win-win situation.

But before I go on, let me give you seven reasons Facebook advertisements work.

1. It's effective.
With billions of user's promoting on Facebook, it's probably more of a guaranteed way to get in front of your ideal client. I am not talking about the organic reach, Facebook will do as you instruct and place your post in front of the person you ask them to. There is no 'fingers crossed' method like there is with organic reach. If your posts are getting good organic reach, and people are commenting and liking them, then Facebook is seeing who is engaging with you. It sees your entertaining and will continue to share your posts. However, if you don't have a good organic reach, and Facebook doesn't think your posts are entertaining or engaging, you have no option but to pay for those posts to get out there.

2. Easy to set up.
Within 10 minutes you can get a simple ad set up, the ads manager makes it an easy process to work through with check boxes and steps. The only hard part is coming up with good, engaging copy.

3. Targets your audience
We spoke about this before, but I feel I must touch on it again, advertisements on Facebook and Instagram means you get access to the 1.6 billion users, with an average person spending up to 50 minutes a day on social media you have a captive audience. Using Facebook ads you'll reach every single one of them.
Facebook has also made it easy, so you can customize your target audiences, based on their interest, demograph-

ics, location, actions on your website, engagement in your app and much more. You can target someone who uses an iPad, likes to read thrillers and lives in New York if you want to.

4. It's cheap
You can literally spend £5 and reach 1,000 people. It makes little sense to spend more, like you would have to do with radio ads, television commercials, billboards, and other traditional media to reach the same audience. Plus, if you missed reason 3, it has targeted those 1000, who are more likely to like your stuff. With other traditional forms of advertising, you are hoping one person watching will connect with your message.

5. It's fast
There are immediate results when you click publish, I have seen results within 2 hours of getting an ad approved. Hitting your audiences timeline, all it requires is for them to click on your ad.

Campaign ID	Campaign name	Result Type	Results	Reach	Impressions	Link clicks	Clicks (all)	Unique link clicks	Landing page views	Social reach
6096084527432	ONE STROKE - JULY18	Landing page views	7	151	151	10	14	10	7	26
6096082201232	NEW TO NAIL ART_JULY18	Landing page views	8	216	217	12	22	12	8	48
6096085569632	event offer- july18	Landing page views		72	72	2	3	2		12
6093852865432	ONE STROKE 2 LAUNCH	Link clicks	3294	34800	62121	3294	4354	3134	2713	9346
				34800	62561	3318	4393	3136	2728	9344

I wanted to show you this report, this was 1 hour after I posted the top three ads on Facebook. You can see already people are clicking through my link and sharing my advert. The final row is an ad I did at the end of June, for 1 week only. You can see how many people I reached and how many people clicked on the ad which ran for just 5 days. Not everyone bought, but I have re-targeted them with the July One Stroke advert, so they will see it again.

6. It's an Investment
Advertise for the express aim to increase brand awareness, spend £10 for 1 week and Target local groups and people in your area to become aware that there is a salon or a service near them. The more familiar people are with your brand, the more likely they will purchase your products when it is time to decide. Follow this up with a flyer through the door. All you need is the return of one service to have paid for the ad. Another option is the "new client call out ad" or the "holiday package offer" there are many ways to get a return on investment, but don't spend more than you think you will get back. Start with £5 for the weekend and work up to £20 for a week. The more you spend the more people you will get in front of.

7. It increases website traffic
Facebook advertising will boost your website traffic. You can run a website click campaign to target your audience and send them to your website. Once they are on your website there is more opportunity for them to sign up to a mailing list, turning your like into a lead. Check out the report above, I had 2713 people visit my website over 5 days.

But I think for most people the hesitation is the cost, what will they get out of it. Facebook advertising is budget-friendly, that means if you want to spend a fiver or 500 on an ad you can. You are in control of your destiny. Now I will not say it will definitely work, there is an art to advertisements on Facebook, and it's not enough to just advertise and hope. Your ad needs to be engaging and have a call to action. The image or video needs to be a scroll stopper.

Basics to Advertising

So this book is not about how to create an ad on Facebook, There will be more on advertising, setting up an advert and what to say in your ad in my new marketing course. You can learn more about that here; https://sam-biddle.co.uk/beinspired/sams-marketing-secrets-course-wait/
You can watch an ad set up and find out more about creating the perfect ad for your audience.

But I want to help clarify a few things and help you understand the world of advertisements and how to get the best from them.

So in this part of the book, I will touch on the basics. There are three main areas you need to understand and master when it comes to advertisements.

1. What type of ad do you need?

There are a few different reasons to place an ad, what is it you're hoping to achieve? I have listed the top six I think are the most effective for salon businesses. It's important to understand the aim of your ad, what do you want someone to do when they click your ad, what's the reason for placing an ad. If it's for more page likes or subscribers, then you would hit the website conversion tab or the page likes tab. There are some which will just help you boost brand awareness, a good thing in my opinion.

Clicks to Website
Clicks to Website ads allow you to link to specific pages on your website in the news feed for both desktop & mobile users and the right sidebar.

Website Conversions
Website Conversions ads allow you to direct visitors to specific pages with the goal of turning those visitors into sales, leads, or subscribers.

Page Post Engagement
Page Post Engagement ads allow you to increase the number of Likes, shares, and comments on your Facebook page posts.
You'll be able to use video, photo, or text ads in the news feed.

.Page Likes
Page Likes ads allow you to target the audiences that'll be most likely to convert into business & encourage them to become fans of your page, although I would always try to do this organically.

Video Views
Video Views ads allow you to drive just that - views to your videos. These ads are optimised by Facebook to be shown to people most likely to watch them.

Offer Claims
Offer Claims ads allow you to drive people to your store using a special offer.

2. How does your advert look?

Think about your Facebook news feed for a second. What does it look like? If I head over to Facebook now, I see a timeline filled with auto-play video's, dozens of pictures, status updates, trending news stories, recommendations, upcoming events and more. That's not including the Facebook Ads I see on both the sidebar and in the news feed. Creating an ad that stands out from the noisy news feed is a tall order.

Will you choose a single ad image, a slideshow, or a video? What's your message and the call to action button? Yes, it is a minefield but here are my six top tips to remember to get the perfect ad.

1. Use a colour that contrasts clearly with the blue and white of the Facebook news feed. Yellow works well and stops that thumb from scrolling.
2. Use simple, clean images with large text on them (20% of image max).
3. Avoid images that have many small details or text and opt for something simple instead. Pets and children work well, but make sure your image relates to what you're offering.
4. Use words like "free," use percentage or money symbols to catch the eye with value.
5. Tell your audience why they need your service in no uncertain terms. Be clear and spell it out.
6. Use customer testimonials and reviews as social proof.

3.Choosing the right audience.

Your Facebook ad will only be effective depending on how well you define your audience.

Now, we have talked a lot already about your target audience and you should know them pretty well already. Their wants, desires, and pain points.

But it now gets interesting, Facebook will let you decide on your audience's demographics. Age, where they live, job and interests, all very important if you want to reach the right person with your ad.

Facebook has made this easy- when you set up your audience you can define them with the user's details, and they give you an idea of the reach you might expect.

The more you hone the details, the more likely your ad is to resonate with users that are interested in what you offer.

4.Video Ads versus images

Video Ads are booming, especially on Facebook where users spend more time watching a video as opposed to text or image-based content.

You can think of a video ad as a mini commercial for your brand. Videos are a great way to stop scrollers in their tracks to see what your ad is about, but this requires putting a video ad together, something I will cover in my marketing course. Learn more here https://sambiddle.co.uk/beinspired/sams-marketing-secrets-course-wait/

We have come to the end of the book, but not to the end of the subject. There is a magic to marketing, but I know it might seem very overwhelming at first. There are so many new things and different ways to doing things that you thought were quite easy.

I get it, trust me, when you have to try and do something new and different it seems like it takes hours away from the things you feel you should be doing. It gets easier, familiar and maybe even exciting.

There is so much more to say on this subject and a lot of things to open up and explore further. It is jolly hard to try and make a book concise, and interesting and not send you to sleep. I hope you have enjoyed this book and found it useful. Please do leave a review if you have purchased this on Amazon, or on my facebook page https://www.facebook.com/beinspired.sambiddle/

If you are interested in my online course please follow this link. https://sambiddle.co.uk/beinspired/sams-marketing-secrets-course-wait/

In the interest of good marketing I shall be adding all my contact details here, so please reach out to me if you have any questions or comments.

Thank you again for buying this book

Sam

Sam Biddle
Be inspired
www.sambiddle.online
www.sambiddle.co.uk
Email beinspired@sambiddle.co.uk

Keep Reading for my bonus chapters on nail art & the reference guide to some of the verbiage in this book.

Reference Guide.

Engagement

When your client or customer directly participate in your marketing, normally through social media. In this book we are looking at the likes, hearts, comments and shares as a form of engagement. A reply to your email is also a client ezgademing with your marketing. The end result is to build a relationship through this engagement.

Organic reach

Organic reach is the total number of people who were shown your post through unpaid distribution. That is the definition as laid out from facebook. The higher the engagement of a post, will also help your organic reach, and means you don't have to spend money getting your message across social media and to your customer.

Paid for reach

Paid reach is the number of people who have seen your post which is a paid post from your Page.

Platform

A Marketing platform is a place which allows you to sell your product or services online. These could be social media, like facebook, instagram, twitter, websites, eBay, Amazon for example.

Content

This is the blurb, words, offers images, video, anything you produce for marketing purposes. This book has content, the words and information on marketing. My online courses have video content. It is what is contained in the thing you are producing at the time.

A lead

A lead is a person's information. It is probably one of the most valuable resources in marketing. As long as you treat them well and with respect. A lead is essentially a person, who has trusted you enough to hand over their contact information.

Audience

Just like the real world an audience is a group of people, but these people are put together based on where they have been, what they like. Your clients will be one audience. The people who visit your website would be an audience. If you do decide to do some paid facebook ads, then you will need to out together an audience of people who you think might want to look at your ad.

ROI

This means your return on investment. Put simply you bought this book for £12, and if using the book's advice you decided to post on Facebook and out of that got 4 new clients each worth £36 each. Your return on investment would be 900%. You can do an online calculation here; https://www.omnicalculator.com/business/roi

To calculate your own ROI; it is the GAIN minus Cost divided by cost which will give you the percentage.

Lead magnet

This is also known as opt-in bribe or an incentive you can offer to potential client in exchange for their contact information such as name, email.

Pain Point

A pain point is a problem, real or perceived that your client might have and you as a marketeer can create opportunities and solutions to help those pain points go away. So if your client has split ends or root growth, that is a pain point which you as a hair stylist can solve. Your client might have badly bitten nails, and as a nail professional you can solve it.

I hope I have included all of the 'sticky' words which have you reaching for google. if not please drop me a line on beinspired@sambiddle.co.uk. I would be happy to answer any of your questions.

Bonus Chapter
Turn inspiration into art.

I could not write a book for beauty and nail professionals and not include nail art, I have popped it at the end as a bonus chapter, as most of you might not be interested in it. However, some points I make could relate to hair and beauty. So it might be worth a quick read through.

Nail art is the backbone of my business, and to be honest with you, this was the first chapter I wrote, when penning this book. It's where I sit most comfortably.

From charging, display and even marketing your nail art this book should help you. But what about the ideas you have in your brain? You know the one that pops open in the middle of the night and you're like yeah that would be awesome. When you come to sit down and create, one of two things happen;

1. You attempt the design and quickly get frustrated and annoyed that what might have looked simple is now looking like a mess on your tip.

2. It is like looking at a blank page, all crisp and white and you have no clue where to start.

Nail art comes in two forms, client-friendly and wild and whacky. But it the Client friendly, wearable nail art we should be interested in, it is salon viable and cost-effective. Don't get me wrong, there is a place for those advanced designs, bringing in interest and some welcome ooh's and ah's from social media and your clients.
But those will not pay the bills.

All is not lost, those nails are there to serve as an example to your clients and peers of the level of your skills. You can then upsell a technique or down sell a simpler look which you can do in 10 minutes or fewer.
Yes, you've guessed it, I am leading you right back to that light bulb moment and how to get that look in your head onto a nail...

You have the potential to create something beautiful and all you feel is the pain, anguish, and a failure. How is nail art looking to you now? Fun right?

So here are my top tips to getting those ideas onto your nail canvases.

It is all about planning and prep, gathering your scrapbook of images and ideas. Via Pinterest, a folder on your computer, old school it and cut and paste onto a board. I use Trello for larger projects but Pinterest works well as an instant source of inspiration at your fingertips.

Once you have gathered, collected and cooed over your fellow peers work, you need to separate and organise them into folders.

For example;
- Ombre nail art
- Marble nail art
- Negative space
- Dots
- Flowers
- Holiday nails
- French with twists

You get my drift right? Placing similar designs together in a board, you're distinguishing between the techniques and breaking down the nail art into 3 defined steps of the building.

So the first step to building a new design.

Step 1.
Colour-I always start with a colour - generally, this is the only input my client has - and then add the other contrasting or complimenting colours around this first choice. Don't think about design or look at this point, because it is the colour which should be your guide.

Step 2.
Style-choose what you will use, dots, lace? Use your references to inspire you, your folders are all set up, so it is as simple as scrolling.

Step 3.
Never have the original out in front of you. You need to check it out and memorise it but don't copy it. Copying is bad, don't limit yourself by copying, it will stunt your growth so you can't develop your own style because you will compare yourself to the original all the time. The person who created the original piece did it from a different perspective. They might have had different training and created their own style.

You will also Limit your design because you're concentrating on "recreating" and not giving your "inner artist" room to spread her wings. Copying puts you in a cage!

You end up with tunnel vision! You will always look for "nail art" to copy and not outside inspiration to develop your own sense of style.

- Using someone else's ideas and improving them is ok.
- Being inspired by the artwork and creating your own version is fine.
- Developing a look based on a mixture of images is cool!

So what if you want to do something more than regular salon viable Nail art?

Your references are all around you, it takes a simple Google search of fairies or butterflies to come back with a host of beautiful images which are not on a nail. Then it is up to you to break it down into shapes

,
> The one thing that will stop you will be not starting.
> Now you have your idea in front of you-start…
> Don't THINK, PLAN, PONDER anymore about it….

Allow all the learning to flow, and just start, you can not see what your design will look like, because you have never done it before, so stop trying to look for that finished image in your head. Enjoy the process and just start!

Bonus Chapters
Turn glitter into cash.

There is an age old issue when it comes to talking about nail art, it is not worthwhile; it is not profitable, no one wants it. There are nail technicians who sneer at the mention of nail art and then there are nail techs whose whole reason for doing this job is nail art. Yes, I am that nail tech.

When I started in the nail business some while ago now (yes, you got me, my total denial of the actual time I have spent filing fingernails and polishing toes). Well, way back then there were two schools of thoughts, the nail tech who did nail art and the nail tech who did Pink and Whites. Back then there wasn't any social media, the industry was not the close-knit family it is today, and we had to battle to get our clients to see that nail art was a good thing.

Now as a nail tech who loves nail art, no I shall re-phrase, as an artist who does nails I have figured out just how to get my glitter on those tiny talons and cash in on it too.

Today I spend a lot of my time with my students online, helping and mentoring them to build a bigger and better business in nails, so they can have the luxury of being creative and still pay the mortgage. I want that for you too.

So my nail friend here are my sexy little secrets to turning your glitter into cash, taking those pots of joy out of the drawer and sharing them with the world.

Do the Work!

It is so easy to see something on social media and think to yourself- awwwww I can't possibly do that! Dismiss it and scroll on up the timeline to find something more manageable. Now I would suggest to everyone out there looking at other peoples art, Never copy! Not just because it is a horrible thing to do, but you're sure to fail. You see with every little brush stroke and dot that has gone into a nail design; it has come from the person's heart and projects their experiences and memories. You could not possibly recreate this and get the same 'feeling' from your work.

This is a great thing because it allows someone's work to inspire you and then trust that your own inner creativity will take that inspiration and make it your own.

Without doing the work, without creating nail art you will have nothing to show your clients, you will have nothing to motivate them to have nail art.

Understanding you don't have to recreate someone else's looks, instead, by building on their design and making it your own will help build confidence in your work.

One thing I hear a lot is, I don't have time to do nail art, or it's playtime. So, let's put this a different way. For every hour you spend building your portfolio of designs, could earn you £50 to £100, would you make more time for it?

You see if you charged a client £5 for some nail art and in one month you had 10 people spend the extra £5 or £6 with you, you would pay for your time and gain more in the process.

1. Experience and confidence in your skills and application
2. New income stream
3. Awareness for your salon, because people will walk out of your door with nail art, a guaranteed draw.
4. Something to keep your clients talking and thinking about you
5. Further opportunities to work with nail art outside of the salon, in the industry and competitions.

But it all starts with a few hours set aside a month, to practice your craft, build your design portfolio and decide what to offer your clients next month.

Time management

So you don't have time to create nail art for clients? I understand this, and if my client wanted me to draw roses and fairies on every nail, with only 10 minutes before my next client, I would agree there is no time for that level of design.

We are creative and visual people, and we see some fabulous nail art on Pinterest and want to create it for our clients but this is not always practical. Don't be put off by the time you THINK it will take.

It has been known for me to do crazy elaborate designs before; it is not because I work fast; it is because I have found shortcuts and bent the rules a little to save time.
But there are two things you need to understand about nail art for your clients;
Client friendly nail art means quick, simple and manageable. Think about nail art as a business opportunity, you might not like doing the simple things and yearn to embellish the nail with diamonds and pearls but those designs are luxury. You want to find designs which are short, fast and effective.

Your clients also don't want to spend hours in the chair whilst you finesse their fingernails. She is perfectly happy with a couple of dots and an ombre or two. Over the years I have figured there are two types of nail art. Nail art for the client and nail art for the nail tech.

Trust me, you got this!

You know what colour to use; you know how to draw a line with a brush, you even know how to add glitter, so you've got this! Don't stop yourself offering nail art because you don't think you're good enough or don't feel confident in applying a complicated rose. Start at the beginning, just like everyone else, and if that is two lines and a sweet little ombre so be it. You can't build a house without foundations and those foundations come first, just like the basic fundamentals of nail art. Education is your friend, however, you learn, in class, online or on your own trust that with each lesson you watch, each nail design you study is growing your creativity.
Often when someone tells me they don't offer nail art in the salon because people don't want it, it is more of a case that the tech doesn't want it, they can't do it or don't have the confidence to try it.

It starts with a simple ombre, or a change of colour placement, maybe a gem or two. Stamping is a good place to start because it gives you the lines to colour in. Everything you do for the first time will always challenge you, but you are the only person stopping you, never let fear of failure prevent you from trying.

Display & Inspire

It is important to inspire your clients; they don't know what's going on in your head or how a design might look based on a few Pinterest images you have seen. Take the time to build a range of designs each month and display them. I am going to go into more detail about charging in the next couple of chapters, as I feel it is really important, but I want to introduce you to the psychology of inspiring your clients.

Imagine if each month you add 5 new designs to that board, Those 5 designs could be seasonal, follow a trend or just be something random. Display the 'looks' over ten different tips, so your client can visualise the design, and mentally wear them. Each time she visit's she will be attracted to the display and start to 'look' for something they can imagine wearing.

Now here is the key, put the price next to the nail design. Most people dismiss something they think will be expensive, and will not even mention it for fear of 'being sold to.' But if you marked the row of tip with the small added extra - NOT THE FULL COST WITH THE SERVICE! They can see, it might be a tempting and affordable add on. You have their undivided attention for 90 minutes, to chat and discuss the possibilities, with a visual cue and your encouragement, they may be tempted to purchase.

The reason we don't put a full-service price on there is that we don't want to scare them off with a big number. Say their treatment with you would cost them £40 before they left the house this morning they had spent that money and can expect your service to cost that much. So if you place a tempting nail design with a price tag of £43, they will be like whoa, really that much?
Instantly they will say no, and that is before you have explained. It is much harder to change someone from a No to a Yes. So just £3 next to ten tiny canvases of glorious nail art is a bargain. An easy up-sell!

Think of the benefits of having your nail art walking around the town for the next month. Is spending those 5 or 10 minutes worth the extra interest your nail art could spark.

Make sure they see your board, point out your brand new designs if you make it a habit to change each month then they will have a new view to tempt them every time they come in. Now they might not have it, they may not take you up on the offer of snowmen on the ring fingers but don't panic, they will be AWARE you offer it! What does that mean? When Mary Jones, next has coffee with Sarah Smith, and they chat about nails and hair, you know Mary will tell Sarah how amazing your designs are and how fabulously talented her nail tech is. What does that mean for you? Sarah might not be in a position for nail art and nails but the word has spread and her friend Veronica thinks it is right up her ally. Boom you have a brand new client. Never underestimate the power of recommendation, sometimes it comes from those who just observe.

Bonus Chapters
Mistakes nail artist make

Are you are leaving a lot of money on the table by not tapping into a hidden source of revenue? It only takes a few words, 'I could make your nails more interesting' to open the door to nail art and put £££ in your bank account. Don't worry if they say no, what have you got to lose if you would not ask them in the first place? Up selling if your a nail tech beauty therapist or hair stylist will change your turnover considerably. If 6 people all spent an extra £2 a day with you, over the course of a week that's £72. Over a year that amounts to an additional £3,744. Not bad for stepping outside of your comfort zone.

Another major mistake nail artists make is not listening to the less is more rule. This has not been more appropriate in the world of nail art. It is one of the biggest mistakes I see nail artists make and so I tell my students to KISS the nail, "Keep it simple sexy". So why do we pile on the glitz and glamour?

The main reason is a lack of confidence. You complete a design and then think, "Wow that didn't take long, and it was way too easy, it is obviously not good enough, I mean I didn't break a sweat and get all stressed about it," "I can't charge her for something which didn't make me uncomfortable, I know I will add two roses, ooh and a gem would look good. Ah I know, I have this cool glitter."

Suddenly your client is walking out of the door with £20 worth of nail art and 30 minutes of your time. Just because it didn't take you long or tax your creative brain. Value your worth, every class, online workshop and educational video you have taken has gone into that nail. The tools and materials you have bought is part of the price and the time and practice you have done are worth more than a few £. Know when to stop!

Is your lack of confidence affecting what you offer?

"I can't think of what to do when someone asks for nails" or "My hands shake when someone asks for nail art" is this you? Why does this happen? Because suddenly you have doubting Della on your shoulder telling you-you're not good enough and you can't Be Creative. My friend, she is not real, and she is just there to stop you from taking a step into the unknown. She does not want you to make a mistake or to fail, so she stops you from doing anything in the first place. Here is the truth, your client knows a lot less than you about nails and nail art. If she could paint a nail or create an ombre with pigments, she would not be sat across from you! Right? So, with this in mind, take a breath and trust you've got this, you have the information there in your mind, just let it flow out. Remember, keep the nail art simple, don't overcrowd the design and the rule of 3's.

Copying.

With a world of Pinterest, Instagram and YouTube videos are full of nail art ideas and tutorials, it is difficult to come up with something original and unique. Especially if you think you have no imagination. But by copying someone else's designs, you are destroying any creative juices that might be flowing. The energy it takes to work out how someone came up with something or to figure out why yours doesn't look like theirs is soul destroying and kills any creativity. Remember these looks, tutorials are there to show you how amazing they are, they don't teach you the technique or application secrets.

So here is how you use those tutorials and inspiration images to your advantage. When you see a design or tutorial, instead of wondering how they are doing the design, think about the way you could improve it. Would you change the colours, would you take out one element, would you use this technique combined with another 'look' you saw? You're upgrading the inspiration to something of your own. You're using the nail image or video to inspire you. So stop copying, take someone's design and improve it.

Using the Rule of 3.

No more than 3 colours, no more than 3 subjects, applications or methods and no more than 3 looks on a combo nail design. I have a whole module in my The Inspired for Life course about the rule of 3. Pairing your design down to make it crisp, clean and cohesive is a skill most nail artists fail to grasp. But learning the rule of 3, well it will take your nail art to the next level.

No show, no sell.

So you have attended a course or working through an online nail art course like The Inspired for Life, and your skills and confidence are improving. Do your clients know about this? Have you got a 'show off board up on your nail desk? If you want to make extra money with nail art, learn to share and sell. So every month you take an A4 acrylic leaflet display stand, change the colour of the card to suit your looks and apply 3 rows of new designs with blue tac on the plastic. (You could use an A5 display stand if you have little space in the salon) The trick is to change these nail designs each month. So every time your clients come in she has something new to look at. Now I am not talking about rows and rows of individual nail tip's all with something different. Theme your rows in colour or design. For example, someone can do a simple Ombre 10 times, to create a row.

1. This gives your client an idea of how it might look over ten nails, especially if you represent the size of the tips to the size of the fingernails, pinkies would be a smaller size, etc.
2. It gives your clients the options to choose because each tip would be a different colour combination. So she can be visually inspired and decide whilst she is having her service.
3. Now you can upsell this nail art without even asking. Next to the row of nail tips, have a small price tag of £3 (or more depending on where you are). This would be the add on price. NEVER include the service onto the nail art price because your client would instantly make a negative decision. She might not realise she is already giving you the service price, anyway. So only include the upsell cost. £3 is nothing, a cup of coffee, which she is getting from you for free anyway.

Season your looks, each month it changes, so Halloween would have more scary art and Christmas more festive.

Bonus Chapters
Charging your worth.

The one thing I hear repeatedly is nail artists not charging for nail art.

If you go to a restaurant, order a meal and drink, then decide at the last minute you fancy dessert, when the bill comes you're like - sure yes I ate that cheesecake, happy to pay £5 for it.

You're not like - whoa... I thought it was for free.

Because you know the ingredients need to be paid for, the time to prep, the cost of electric to store and the wages to pay the staff, the cost of training to become a chef... blah blah blah, it all mount's up, so every bite will cost you

Believe it or not, your customer also thinks the same thing.

THERE ARE 3 COMMON REASONS NAIL TECHS DON'T CHARGE.

1. You're taking care of their purse strings instead of your own. You think they won't pay for nail art, but have you even asked?

2. You're worried about not being good enough to charge your worth.

3. You don't have the time to add it on, so you Don't Push It...

So that extra £5 added onto the bill in the restaurant, they took a max of 15 minutes per person to prep and deliver the cheesecake, if there are 50 people a week ordering it that's £250.00 extra. Can you really not afford to promote a simple, fast and effective nail art?

Here is a quick how-to guide.

Find 5 designs which are fast and effective (pigment ombre, nail art pen swirls, stamping) make sure you can do them within 15min... no longer. This will also stop that "my mind is blank, I don't know what to do" situation. Like a Menu, it is all prepared for you in advance.

Create a row of 10, using the same technique and display on a board (keep it simple) in a row, but change up the colour combo. Have all 5 on display on your nail desk. The row of 10, will give your clients a visual of what it would look like over 10 nails and a chance for you to practice and get your speed up.

Add a small price tag (like a menu) net to each design say £3, £5, or £7. NEVER include the price of the service, just the addon... keep it low and affordable.

Wear one of the designs and make sure you ask every client if she would like something extra today. Don't worry if she says no, you have planted a seed.

If she is on the fence, say, I will do two fingers for free (ring finger manicure) if she decides to just stick with that, don't charge, but tell her next time she will want more. Why? Because all her friends will comment.

When she comes back, make sure you ask her how the nail art went, show her the NEW set of 5 designs you have prepared for her. Yes, you will need to change your display each month, so every time your client returns you have more options.

It comes down to money.

We want to get down with the earning potential of nail art. How much do you charge? Now no matter what country I visit, or whom I am talking to, this is the question I can't answer.

Different countries have different pricing, you need to be in line with your competition, but also make sure you covering your overheads and making a profit.

I always tell people they should first work out their own hourly rate. Base this on your costs, materials and time to do one set of nails (include the heating, electric, advertising, staff, and telephone) so to do this, you work out how much it takes to stay open every day.

> Calculate all your costs, overheads and outgoings for the month. Divide this by the amount of days your open and working. Then you have how much you need to earn to stay open each day. Your overheads should include your drawings also.

> Now you have your daily rate, divide this by the number of hours you work, now you have a base rate, this is the rate you NEVER go below. If you want to grow your business and make a profit, you will need to either double it or multiply this rate by 20% or 30%.

> Now you have an hourly rate, we need to divide this by 60, so we have a rate per minute.

You see if you keep the nail art simple so it takes only 10 minutes (15 max) your going to increase your cash flow. You will also keep the cost low enough to make it affordable for the clients and maximise profit. Yes, it might mean adding extra time to your client's appointment, but with a little shuffle around, this is actually a money saver. Starting and stopping a client is dead time, no earning potential. So if you can keep your client there a little longer, you can be earning.

So if your nail art takes you 5 minutes, and you know your rate by the minute, you multiply the two figures together and find out what you need to charge.

Example

- Your hourly rate is £35
- 35 divided by 60 (minutes) =.58p
- If you take 5 minutes to do a design
- 58p x 5 (minutes) = £2.90
- The cost of your design is £2.90

Be Sensible, you might need to round up or round down that figure to make it attractive.

the end

Notes

Notes

Notes

Notes